SpringerBriefs in Psycholog

SpringerBriefs present concise summaries of cutting-edge research and practical applications across a wide spectrum of fields. Featuring compact volumes of 50 to 125 pages, the series covers a range of content from professional to academic. Typical topics might include:

- A timely report of state-of-the-art analytical techniques
- A bridge between new research results as published in journal articles and a contextual literature review
- A snapshot of a hot or emerging topic
- An in-depth case study or clinical example
- A presentation of core concepts that readers must understand to make independent contributions

SpringerBriefs in Psychology showcase emerging theory, empirical research, and practical application in a wide variety of topics in psychology and related fields. Briefs are characterized by fast, global electronic dissemination, standard publishing contracts, standardized manuscript preparation and formatting guidelines, and expedited production schedules.

More information about this series at http://www.springer.com/series/10143

Patricia J. Robinson

Basics of Behavior Change
in Primary Care

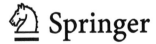 Springer

Patricia J. Robinson
Mountainview Consulting Group, Inc.
Portland, OR, USA

ISSN 2192-8363   ISSN 2192-8371   (electronic)
SpringerBriefs in Psychology
ISBN 978-3-030-32049-2   ISBN 978-3-030-32050-8   (eBook)
https://doi.org/10.1007/978-3-030-32050-8

This Springer imprint is published by the registered company Springer Nature Switzerland AG
The registered company address is: Gewerbestrasse 11, 6330 Cham, Switzerland

To all people on our big blue marble, may you learn to flourish.
Patti Robinson, Wheeler, Oregon, June, 2019

The Purpose of This Book

I am writing this book to help people who want to help others be effective agents of change in the powerful setting of primary care. Primary care is the place where most people can access the services of a healthcare clinician, and this book aims to empower those clinicians to promote changes in behavior that help people to flourish (Fledderus, Bohlmeijer, Smit, & Westerhof, 2010). Whether you are a trained professional and relocating to the primary care setting or a student preparing for a career in primary care, my hope is that this book will help you become an effective member of an interprofessional team, capable of delivering interventions for patients of all ages for all behaviorally influenced problems when the patient asks for help.

I have met and worked with physicians, nurse practitioners, physician assistants, team nurses and nursing assistants, pharmacists, physical therapists, social workers, psychologists, counselors, community healthcare workers, and health coaches all over the world. I have worked in rural, urban, and suburban settings in the United States and provided training and technical assistance in Sweden, Norway, Denmark, France, Spain, Italy, Great Britain, Germany, Ireland, Mexico, Argentina, Canada, Japan, Korea, Australia, Peru, and New Zealand. Everywhere, there are difficulties with healthcare and opportunities for improvement. The ability to effectively support behavior change among patients presenting with medical and psychological problems is central to realizing the *Quadruple Aim* outcomes of improved population health, patient experience, value, and primary care staff wellness (Bodenheimer & Sinsky, 2014).

More and more countries are waking up to this idea and are initiating efforts to make delivery of behavior change services a routine part of primary care. Strategies recommended by the *Primary Care Behavioral Health* (PCBH) model (Reiter, Dobmeyer, & Hunter, 2017; Robinson & Reiter, 2016, 2007) offer guidance for these pilots and large-scale deployment following successful pilots. Dozens of studies on the PCBH model document its promise as an effective population health approach to delivery of behavioral health services and its association with positive clinical and system-level outcomes (Hunter et al., 2017). Strategies in this book are consistent with the PCBH approach, where many more people access behavioral health services than was possible in traditional soloed approaches to healthcare.

PCBH services are also associated with the achievement of health equity, such that people who need healthcare the most can access it as easily as those with better health (www.tetumuwaiori.com).

The most significant barrier to PCBH deployment is the lack of a trained workforce, capable of delivering empirically supported behavior change interventions. This book is an attempt to promote rapid uptake of assessment and intervention strategies by all members of the interprofessional teams that are developing in primary care clinics around the world. This is a small book, with five chapters that can be read in any order by any member of the primary care team. The first chapter introduces readers to primary care—its mission and methods and its current challenges. The second chapter concerns the development and maintenance of strong teams. In the third chapter, I suggest a conceptualization for assisting patients of any age with ongoing development of skills that promote flourishing and healthy aging. Chapter 3 introduces Contextual Interview Questions, a tool that helps clinicians complete a functional assessment of the problem that most concerns the patient. In Chap. 5, readers learn to intervene to promote more psychologically flexible behavior in patients and to develop engaging behavioral experiments with patients. Several metaphors commonly used by PC teams using *Focused Acceptance and Commitment Therapy* (FACT) are introduced, including the Bull's-Eye and the Life Path. Both of these interventions can be used in individual and group visits with patients.

The Appendices offer readers a Contextual Behavioral Scientist Checklist (Appendix A) to track their progress in developing skills in using the toolkit offered by this book. For convenience in duplicating and use of tools and skill practice worksheets, other appendices provide copies of forms introduced in Chaps. 2–5 (including outcome measures in Appendix B, assessment methods in Appendix C, and worksheets in Appendix D). Readers will find these scales and tools on the book website as well (basicsofbehaviorchangeinprimarycare.com).

This book is for all healthcare professionals working to improve health in their communities, including Primary Care Clinicians (PCCs), nursing staff and nursing assistants, Pharmacists (Ph), Physical Therapists (PTs) and their assistants, Behavioral Health Clinicians (BHCs) and their assistants, Dieticians, Emergency Department and Hospital Staff, Specialty Service Providers, Health Coaches (HCs), and Community Health Workers (CHWs). This book is also written for clinic and healthcare system leaders. A fully informed leadership supports rapid, efficient change toward delivery of better primary behavioral healthcare services. To encourage the use of this book by leaders, I include a section for leaders at the end of each chapter (*Tips for Leaders*) as a part of the chapter summary. Knowledge gained from reading this book is a first step toward developing an evolved primary care service; mastery develops as a part of a flexible application of methods and strategies introduced in the book. To encourage our readers to attain mastery, I offer online coaching services to readers seeking assistance in applying and refining what they learned from reading this book (see book website: basicsofbehaviorchangeinprimarycare.com).

Whether you are a healthcare leader or provider or a student preparing for a career in primary care, this book is for you. I hope that students of nursing, psychology, social work, counseling, marriage and family therapy, pharmacy, physical therapy, nutrition, exercise science, epidemiology, public health, and medicine will read this book early in their studies. This book is also for the faculty members that teach them. Increasingly, faculty members will team-teach interdisciplinary courses to graduate and undergraduate students embarking on careers in healthcare. In this way, we develop a group of healthcare providers for the future, one that knows how to deliver high-impact behavior change services as a part of an interprofessional team.

I want to express my gratitude for the many people that assisted with and inspired this book. First, I want to thank Jeff Reiter for mulling over ideas for the book with me and for providing helpful feedback on several chapters. I wish his life circumstances had allowed him to cowrite with me, as he is an excellent writer and a deep thinker. Second, I want to thank Justin Kerr for his proof-reading and editorial assistance; this book would not have been possible without his resolute assistance in the final days of writing. Sharon Penulla, an editor at Springer, has shared a vision of better behavioral health services in primary care with me for almost 15 years. Thank you, Sharon. I also must name a few of my healthcare superheroes, including Kirk Strosahl, Sue Hallwright, Jo Chiplin, Johnny O'Connell, Aaron O'Connell, Marcia Sasano, Julie Geiler, Ann Dobmeyer, Chris Hunter, Neftali Serano, Lt Col Matthew Nelson, Jodi Polaha, Jennifer Funderburk, Katie Kanzler, Kent and Megan Corso, Stacy Ogbeide, Nicola Silberleitner, Anneli Voncederwald, Margaret Lemp, Lisa Braverman, Emily Parker, Julie Oyemaja, Mary Peterson, Robyn Godye, Alysha Simonsen, Emma Usmar, Wayne Blackburn, David Bauman, Bridget Beachy, and Mark Sauerwein. Finally, I am grateful for all the patients that have helped me learn about how to help people make small changes that improve the quality of their lives.

References

Bodenheimer, T., Sinsky, C. (2014). From Triple to Quadruple Aim: Care of the patients requires care of the provider. *Annals of Family Medicine, 12*(6), 573–576. https://doi.org/10.1370/afm.1713

Fledderus, M., Bohlmeijer, E. T., Smit, F., & Westerhof, G. J. (2010). Mental health promotion as a new goal in public mental healthcare: a randomized controlled trial of an intervention enhancing psychological flexibility, *American Journal of Public Health, 100*, 2372–2378. https://doi.org/10.2105/AJPH.2010.196196

Hunter, C. L., Funderburk, J. S., Polaha, J., Bauman, D., Goodie, J. L., & Hunter, C. M. (2017). Primary Care Behavioral Health (PCBH) model research: Current state of the science and a call to action. *Journal of Clinical Psychology in Medical Settings*. https://doi.org/10.1007/s10880-017-9512-0

Reiter, J. T., Dobmeyer, A. C., & Hunter, C. L. (2017). The primary care behavioral health (PCBH) model: An overview and operational definition. *Journal of Clinical Psychology in Medical Settings, 24*(4).

Robinson, P. J., & Reiter, J. D. (2007). *Behavioral consultation and primary care: A guide to integrating services.* New York, NY: Springer.

Robinson, P. J., & Reiter, J. D. (2016). *Behavioral consultation and primary care: A guide to integrating services* (2nd ed.). New York, NY: Springer.

The Alphabet Soup of the Evolving Primary Care Team

This is a list of the most commonly used abbreviations in this book. They include abbreviations for titles of team members and models for delivery of primary care services.

Additionally, each chapter includes a list of the abbreviations used in that chapter.

BHC	Behavioral Health Clinician
BHC-A	Behavioral Health Clinician-Assistant
Dt	Dietician
CHW	Community Health Worker
CL	Clinic Leaders
HC	Health Coach
LPN	Licensed Practical Nurse
LP	Liaison Psychiatric Prescriber
MA	Medical Assistant
PC	Primary Care
PCC	Primary Care Clinician
Ph	Pharmacist
Ph-A	Pharmacist Assistant
PT	Physical Therapist
PT-A	Physical Therapist Assistant
PCBH	Primary Care Behavioral Health
PCMH	Patient Centered Medical Home
RN	Nurse

List of Abbreviations

BHC	Behavioral Health Clinician
CHW	Community Health Worker
FACT	Focused Acceptance and Commitment Therapy
HC	Health Coach
MA	Medical Assistant
PC	Primary Care
PCBH	Primary Care Behavioral Health
PCC	Primary Care Clinician
PT	Physical Therapist
PT-A	Physical Therapist Assistant
PCBH	Primary Care Behavioral Health

Contents

List of Figures

List of Tables

List of Appendices

About the Author

Patricia J. Robinson Patti Robinson, PhD, is the Director of Training and Program Evaluation for Mountainview Consulting Group (www.Mtnviewconsulting.com). This company was founded in 1998 and won the APA Presidential Innovative Practice Award in 2009. Current projects include consulting, training, and writing. Dr. Robinson provides trainings in primary care behavioral health and Focused Acceptance and Commitment Therapy all over the world, including Hong Kong, Sweden, Finland, the Netherlands, Spain, Germany, Italy, Great Britain, Australia, New Zealand, Denmark, Norway, Finland, Italy, and the United States. She is committed to healthcare transformation and to improving care to all people, particularly underserved people. Her interests also include prevention science and use of contextual behavioral science and principles of prosocial group design to enhance clinician resiliency and primary care team effectiveness. Earlier in her career, she worked as a researcher and clinician for Group Health Cooperative in Seattle, WA and as a Behavioral Health Consultant for Yakima Valley Farm Workers Clinic in Toppenish, WA. She has over 50 professional publications, including 11 books.

Chapter 1
Primary Care

Abbreviations

BHC	Behavioral Health Clinician
BHC-A	Behavioral Health Clinician-Assistant
CBT	Cognitive Behavioral Therapy
Dt	Dietician
ED	Emergency Department
EHR	Electronic Health Record
NCQA	National Committee on Quality Assurance
PC	Primary Care
PCBH	Primary Care Behavioral Health model
PCC	Primary Care Clinician
PCMH	Patient Centered Medical Home
PT	Physical Therapist
US	United States

The phrase "form follows function" was suggested by architect Louis H. Sullivan in an 1896 essay, "The Tall Office Building Artistically Considered." This thought-provoking phrase has provoked many discussions among architects over the years. To what extent should the design of something support its function? Frank Lloyd Wright, Sullivan's student, extended Wright's perspective, stating that "form and function are one". This chapter is about the architecture of healthcare and how to build it, so that healthcare functions well and is beautiful to the users and the providers. It includes an introduction to primary care (PC), its mission, and its challenges. Readers will learn about the Triple Aim, the Patient Centered Medical Home (PCMH) model, and the Primary Care Behavioral Health (PCBH) model. We end the chapter with a list of recommended strategies for improving the union of form and function in primary care by enhancing patient access to behavior change services.

P. J. Robinson, *Basics of Behavior Change in Primary Care*, SpringerBriefs
in Psychology, https://doi.org/10.1007/978-3-030-32050-8_1

Form and Function

Primary Care Clinicians (PCCs) deliver primary care services in different forms all over the United States and in other countries as well. The settings for delivery vary greatly, ranging from small solo practice clinics owned by PCCs to large clinics owned by healthcare corporations operating in multiple states. Primary care services are also delivered in schools, daycare units, shopping malls, airports, long-term care units, and in-home care units. In rural, urban, and suburban America, people of all ages, cultures and socioeconomic resources visit PC clinics. A PC clinic is usually the patient's first point of entry into the healthcare system and the focal point for future healthcare needs.

Primary care offers the widest range of services of all healthcare endeavors, and this is consistent with its mission. The Institute of Medicine's definition of PC is clear, and it continues today in wording originally offered in 1996 (Institute of Medicine (US) Committee on the Future of Primary Care, 1996):

> Primary care is the provision of integrated, accessible health care services by clinicians who are accountable for addressing a large majority of personal health care needs, developing a sustained partnership with patients, and practicing in the context of family and community.

The qualities of integrated, accessible, and continuous care for the majority of healthcare needs, and connection with family and community are central to questions of form and function in on-going evolution of PC toward successful realization of its mission.

The work of Barbara Starfield and others have documented the critical importance of PC as the hub of a well-functioning healthcare system. Research shows that countries with the most robust PC have the healthiest populations. The benefits of strong PC include better health outcomes, a more equitable distribution of care, and lower healthcare spending. Unfortunately, the U.S. has not recognized the importance of PC and has built a reimbursement and care delivery system that favors specialty care. This has resulted in ballooning healthcare costs in the United States (US) and contributed to the US ranking lower than many other countries on various key health metrics measured across countries (for more on the above, see Starfield, Shi & Macinko, 2005 and Starfield, 2008).

While responsible for helping patients prevent health problems, develop and maintain strong family relationships, address acute health problems, and manage chronic health conditions, PC has not been funded adequately for delivery of behavioral health services. PCCs see between 15 and 30 patients a day and have little time for recognizing and addressing the role of psychosocial distress in the patient's presentation. Efforts to help patients access social services and to advocate for patients' health needs are often thwarted by lack of resources in the community. This form of PC has not supported the functions of PC and the costs—in human suffering and in dollars—are substantial for individuals, families, communities, governmental agencies at the state and federal level and to the providers of PC. With the inclusion of behavioral health services, provided by all members of a team, PC will work better and better achieve its mission.

Current Initiatives in Primary Care

Healthcare innovators, researchers, and policy makers are continuously striving to define, deploy, and refine primary care operations in order to improve outcomes. The Triple Aim is a common term for describing the core components against which attempts to improve quality are measured. The *Patient Centered Medical Home* (PCMH) offers guidance about how to change primary care operations in order to improve Triple Aim outcomes, and the *Primary Care Behavioral Health* (PCBH) model is a group of strategies for improving patient access to care for medical and behavioral health concerns.

Triple Aim

Berwick, Nolan, and Whittington first described the Triple Aim in 2008. The Triple Aim suggests that there are three key factors in improving healthcare outcomes. These include: (1) improve the patient experience of care, including quality and satisfaction, (2) improve the health of populations, and (3) reduce the per capita cost of healthcare. Siefel and Nolan (2012) offer a guide to Triple Aim measurements. Berwick, Nolan and Whittington's 2008 report noted that despite spending far more than any other country on healthcare services, the U.S. ranks far below other countries on healthcare outcomes. They use care of congestive heart failure, the most common reason for admission of Medicare patients to a hospital, to illustrate problems in the current healthcare system. Almost 40% of patients hospitalized for congestive heart failure are readmitted to the hospital within 90 days, even though well-documented demonstration projects have shown that proper management of patients can reduce the readmission rate by more than 80%. Thus, owing not to a lack of knowledge or technology, but rather to various deficits and inefficiencies in the current system, these patients are not as healthy as they could be, and their care costs more.

Quadruple Aim

Bodenheimer and Sinsky suggested that the Triple Aim be expanded to include the health and well-being of all the people working in PC clinics (Bodenheimer & Sinsky, 2014). As more clinics adopted the Triple Aim, it became clear that stressful work life circumstances were a barrier to achievement of the three aims. A fourth aim was needed, and that aim was to improve the work life of clinicians and staff. Upskilling the PC team in behavior change science has the potential to supercharge their pursuit of all four aims: improving population health, improving patient experience, enhancing value, and promoting primary care staff wellness.

Patient Centered Medical Home Model

The Patient Centered Medical Home (PCMH; also referred to as "Medical Home", "Health Care Home", and "Patient Centered Health Care Home") suggests goals for PC clinics to pursue in order to improve the outcomes of care. The major PC associations joined together to create and publish the *Joint Principles of the Patient Centered Medical Home* in 2007. Since then, the model has evolved to consist of these five components (Agency for Healthcare Research and Quality, 2014):

1. *Comprehensive Care*: The PCMH must meet the majority of a patient's physical and MH care needs, including preventive, acute and chronic care. This is accomplished by building a team of diverse care providers.
2. *Patient Centered*: Care is relationship-based, involving patients as partners, and respecting their culture, values and preferences.
3. *Coordinated Care*: The PCMH should coordinate services provided by specialists, home healthcare workers, hospitals staff, community services workers, and others.
4. *Accessible Services*: A PCMH should have shorter waiting times for appointments, hours that are convenient to the patient, and care team members that are available through a variety of means, including email, healthcare record portals and phone.
5. *Quality and Safety*: The PCMH should engage in continuous quality improvement and use evidence-based care and population health strategies.

In 2011, the *National Committee for Quality Assurance* (NCQA), the primary agency responsible for certifying, or "recognizing," an organization as a PCMH, provided program standards for PCMH clinics. The six standards include: (1) patient-centered access to care; (2) team-based care; (3) population health management; (4) care management and support; (5) tracking and coordination of care (e.g., for referrals); (6) measuring and improving performance. Recognition is voluntary, and the NCQA helps clinics prepare for recognition. Assistance includes ensuring that Electronic Health Records (EHR) systems, advanced registries, population health management tools and other technology related aspects of care align with PCMH standards (AHRQ, 2014).

While many studies conducted in a variety of settings, and even different countries, have shown that the PCMH can improve quality, lower costs, reduce errors, and improve patient satisfaction (for example, see Reid, et al., 2010 and Rosenthal, 2008), the validity of some studies has been questioned. One criticism is that PCMH is often applied very differently from one system to another. Also, some PCMH studies have not been able to replicate the positive findings of other studies (Hoff, Weller & DePuccio, 2012; Peikes, Zutshi, Genevro, Parchman & Meyers, 2012). At this time, many researchers are studying the impact of PCMH relative to the outcomes obtained with standard care. The studies are looking at outcomes for all patients and for patient groups for which outcomes are particularly concerning, such as patients coping with chronic disease. The PCMH model of primary care appears to be more effective than standard care for improving clinical outcomes for patients with chronic disease, but the strength of the evidence base is unclear (John, Ghassempour, Girosi, & Atlantis, 2018).

Unfortunately, the role of a behavioral health provider in primary care was not perceived as essential to improving outcomes by early proponents of PCMH. PCMH policy papers, other than those written by behavioral health professionals, say little about the role of behavioral health providers in PC. A lack of attention to the central importance of a behavioral health provider on the team has contributed to PC clinics conceptualizing the PCMH team as comprised of usual staff, such as the physician, RN, lab technician, and MA. Freeman argues that, "Behaviorists…are considered external to the Healthcare Home by the chief architects of the concept."

The American Psychological Association Practice Association (2009) has also noted this and has lobbied for change. Advocacy for behavioral health providers on the PCMH team has had an impact, as the 2014 revision of the PCMH standards do promote enhanced care for behavioral issues; however, they still do not require a *Behavioral Health Clinician* (BHC) be integrated into the team.

Given that so much of what the PCMH is intended to help with involves conditions with a behavioral component, the lack of attention to inclusion of a team member with expertise in behavior change has quite possibly slowed progress toward achievement of the Quadruple Aim. This is supported by data from a Blue Cross/ Blue Shield analysis of care outcomes in the PCMH of Cherokee Health Systems, in Tennessee, which do include a BHC (Freeman, 2011). Specifically, the study compared patients from the behaviorally enhanced Cherokee PCMH to standard care patients in the same region of Tennessee. Cherokee patients used emergency rooms, medical specialists, and hospital care significantly less; and the overall cost of Cherokee's patients was significantly and substantially lower.

Given the behavioral nature of so many of the problems seen in PC, the PCMH team that adds a BHC will most likely move more swiftly toward the Quadruple Aim. However, the impact of adding a BHC to PC without training the BHC and other team members and without making changes to workflows may be of limited value. A move to integrate a BHC requires that the PCMH team follow the guidance of an established model. We turn our attention now to a brief description of that model.

Primary Care Behavioral Health Model

The Primary Care Behavioral Health (PCBH) model provides instructions for integrating a BHC into PCMH clinics, and standard care clinics as well (Reiter, Dobmeyer, & Hunter, 2017; Robinson & Reiter, 2015, 2007). The PCBH mission is to improve healthcare outcomes—clinical, cost/value, patient and provider experience—by assuring availability of services informed by behavioral science to all patients at the time of their need. A recent review of 29 studies on the PCBH model found that it shows promise as an effective population health approach to behavioral health service delivery and that it is associated with positive patient and implementation outcomes (Hunter et al., 2017).

The PCBH model brings a *Behavioral Health Clinician* (BHC) to clinics to work as a *fully integrated* team member. The staffing ratio for BHCs is usually one for every three to five thousand patients, with the panel size smaller for clinics serving patients with greater complexity. The BHC works as a generalist, seeing patients of any age for brief visits (30 minutes at the most) designed to focus on the problem of concern for the patient and to improve the patient's ability to function in important life roles, including that of having a meaningful connection with family and community, the experience of satisfaction in one's day-to-day endeavors, and the skills to maintain good health. BHCs also work with colleagues in developing multidisciplinary pathways that target patient groups whose health outcomes are problematic. The BHC shifts from a traditional mental health therapist role to that of a consultant that provides "a little behavioral health intervention for a lot of patients". The BHC attempts to teach their new colleagues to use new skills to promote behavior change and to thereby attain better outcomes. Additionally, the BHC attempts to assist with development of new practice management habits and realization of greater efficiency in daily work. The BHC partners with quality improvement staff in efforts to assess processes and outcomes important to successful delivery of integrated services. The BHC also aligns with clinic leaders responsible for developing and monitoring a business plan for integrated care. Being an effective BHC requires a large set of skills, and most BHCs only acquire these skills over years of practice and on-going study and mentoring from BHCs with greater experience.

The PCBH model also provides guidance about small changes to the roles and responsibilities of staff and modification of workflows as a clinic transitions to PCBH status. To facilitate an optimal change process, clinic leaders and all staff members receive brief, on-the-job training in new competencies (see Robinson & Reiter, 2015 for core competency tools for BHCs, PCCs, and RNs; see Robinson, Oyemaja, Beachy, Goodie, Sprague, Bell, Maples, & Ward, 2018 for a competency tool for clinic leaders).

PCBH competency tools require trainees to develop a strong knowledge base and the abilities to (1) consistently demonstrate use of specific clinical and practice management skills, (2) demonstrate consistent practice of strong documentation habits, (3) develop and evaluate programs to improve healthcare outcomes, (4) meet productivity standards and (5) work effectively as a member of a team, demonstrating work habits that bring a source of satisfaction and meaning to their career experience and to the experience of their teammates.

Because of both the demonstrated and expected benefits of inclusion of BHCs on PCMH teams, healthcare funders in the US are beginning to offer incentives to PCMH sites that offer BHC services. The primary barrier to widespread rapid transition of PCMH clinics to behaviorally enhanced clinics is the lack of a trained behavioral health workforce ready to work as PC BHCs. There are a small and growing group of veteran BHCs available to assist clinics in implementing PCBH strategies, including recruiting and training BHC team members. There is also a PCBH manual template available for clinics (see https://www.MtnviewConsulting.com.).

The primary purpose of this book is to provide a common approach to behavioral assessment and intervention so that all members of behaviorally enhanced PCMH teams work together to address the healthcare needs of all primary care patients for all health challenges.

Challenges to Evolving Primary Care

Even with the helpful structure provided by the Quadruple Aim and the PCMH and PCBH models, primary care faces many challenges to providing healthcare services with a strong behavioral and social focus. These challenges include clinician and system factors and they are interwoven and difficult to unravel and re-shape. Therefore, change may not come quickly, and healthcare innovators will need great skill in communicating and working in small groups with persistence. With these qualities, change will come, one small step at a time. Let's take a look at the challenges, with a goal of identifying opportunities for improvement.

Lack of Preparation

In many universities, the students who will become the healthcare providers of tomorrow train in different departments, perhaps never meeting people who will be their teammates when they move into primary care. For many disciplines, the training provided on behavioral science is off-the-mark for working in the real world of primary care. For example, medical students may have behavioral scientists in their residency practice that model the skill for conducting hour long interviews with families. Though interesting and important in its own right, most PCCs will never have time to spend an hour with a family. Instead, they will complete 20 or more 15-minute visits with patients with wide-ranging medical, psychological and social problems every day. Rarely, would a student aspiring to be a pharmacist learn about the principals of behavior modification and methods of functional analysis, although such would certainly empower the effectiveness of a clinical pharmacists. Most students of physical therapy and nursing do not receive training in how to help patients clarify their values related to health or to train their attention so that more intentional health-promoting choices are possible. Most of these students will learn about psychopathology and diagnostic criteria for common disorders, and, unfortunately, these skills may not contribute to their ability to engage patients in services that teach patients the skills they need to live more meaningful lives.

Similarly, current professional trainings for today's licensed healthcare providers tend to focus on diagnosis, use of medications, and monitoring of symptoms of psychopathology. These trainings connect well with healthcare providers whose original training was in a biomedical rather than a biopsychosocial model. They do not help the clinician expand their skills or shift their perspective to a biopsychosocial model where they might better engage patients and experience greater success in their clinical work. A look at continuing education courses offered at annual conventions for mental health clinicians reveals numerous options for learning more lengthy psychotherapies and time-intensive testing procedures and relatively fewer options on brief treatment, teamwork, and primary care behavioral health.

Cognitive Behavioral Therapy (CBT) is a cost-effective approach to behavior change, that could be used by a diverse group of professionals; however, most do not receive training due to cost or perhaps the perception that the treatment is complex and too time-intensive. The result is that most patients with a mental health disorder do not receive an evidence-based intervention, and, sadly, most don't receive any treatment. Better preparation for healthcare providers of today and tomorrow is certainly a challenge, but one that must be addressed.

Low Job Control

Another challenge to the typical healthcare provider's efforts to better address the behavioral health needs of their patients is that of problematic *job control*, or limited ability to influence what happens in the work environment. Ratings on measures of job control indicating higher levels of control are associated with higher levels of job satisfaction. When one lacks options for influencing the way they complete their work, they experience stress and if this persists, stress can develop into a sense of demoralization. This is particularly true when a lack of control relates closely to personal values and goals. Most people who go into healthcare truly value helping others, and they perceive the important role that psychological and social factors play in healthcare outcomes. Unfortunately, these well-intentioned clinicians may work in a clinic that emphasizes quantity and experience a conflict between a need to meet productivity standards at the cost of working more closely with patient needs. Clinicians may experience lowered job control in areas other than their ability to provide comprehensive biopsychosocial care, such as use of electronic healthcare records that are complex, non-intuitive and unreliable. All workplace factors that lower job control sum together and when that sum is high the clinician may begin to lose a strong personal connection with the values that brought them to healthcare in the first place.

High Complexity Patients

More complex patients have more medical and behavioral health problems, but most clinics do not allow PCCs more time to address these problems. Further, PCCs may be paid for addressing medical problems but not for addressing behavioral health problems. When working in traditional clinics, PCCs may not be able to shift some of the work to teammates or access electronic support for on-going monitoring and delivery of patient care. All too often, the results lead to complex patients becoming sicker and needing more services which are often costly services such as emergency department (ED) and hospital services. PCCs again may feel at a loss to reverse the patient's cycle from disability to ability without new skills and new teammates.

Workforce Shortage

There is a shortage of PC physicians and this shortage will grow in the immediate future for a variety of reasons. Aging and population growth will increase demand for healthcare in the future, with older adults soon comprising one in five people in America. People over 65 make about three times as many healthcare visits as people in their thirties. Another factor that influences the growth of the workforce shortage is the aging of physicians, with an increasingly large number of physicians moving into retirement age in the next decade. While this might be addressed by creating more physicians, many new physicians chose a sub-specialty like cardiology or plastic surgeon where their salary will be twice that of what a primary care physician earns. This is a significant factor given the student loans that physicians incur during the typical 10-year period of training. The shortage may contribute to a focus on training physicians to focus on medical care rather than take a more wholistic view where behavior change is on equal footing with biological concerns.

Recommended Strategies for Improving Behavioral Health Services in Primary Care

To assist readers in imagining ways to address the challenges to enhancing delivery of behavior change services in primary care, we offer nine strategies. These strategies are listed in Checklist of Strategies for Improving Delivery of Behavioral Health Services in Primary Care (Table 1.1). Some will pay more dividends in some communities than others, so guidance in this section includes the identification of contextual factors in the community that may influence the viability and necessity of the strategies.

1. *Build a team*: Teamwork is a powerful strategy for addressing multiple challenges, including job control and burnout. Members of a well-trained team are capable of implementing biopsychosocial care efficiently and consistently. In Chap. 2, we provide information about possible new members of a primary care team that can help address the behavioral healthcare needs of healthy patients, patients with chronic disease, and patients facing the trials of aging. We also suggest strategies for creating and maintaining healthy relationships among teammates and principals for creating teams that produce the best outcomes given the resources available to the team. Of course, available resources vary from clinic to clinic. Some clinics have many resources while others have few. Roles and

responsibilities of team members vary according to resources and resources, even within a clinic, vary from time to time.

2. *Use team-based metrics*: Historically, all of the responsibility for outcomes has fallen upon the physician in charge of the team. While understandable, this arrangement places a great deal of pressure upon the physician and misses the mark in terms of enlisting the optimal involvement of all team members in pursuing the best outcomes for patients and for the team. Metrics that reflect the work of the team encourage each team member to be fully involved in the work of the team on an on-going basis. The work of the team takes priority over the work of the individual and with this shift there is an opportunity for increased cooperation and efficiency. An example of a team metric is that of cycle time. Clinic visit cycle time is the amount of time in minutes that a patient spends at an office visit. The cycle begins at the time of arrival and ends when the patient leaves the clinic. Many team members are involved in managing cycle time and this type of metric can be used to enhance patient experience, particularly if all team members are rewarded for contributing to lowering cycle time. An additional aspect of team-based metrics worthy of mention is that of involvement of all team members in creating and prioritizing strategies for pursuit of team metrics. It may be a nursing assistant that offers the best idea for addressing a problem. Every team member has their own perspective and all perspectives are important. Asking and valuing the ideas of all team members creates a feeling of workplace autonomy, which is in some ways the opposite of low job control.

3. *Use assistants and extenders more*: It takes 10 years to train a physician and about the same amount of time to train a psychologist. Physical therapists, dieticians, social workers, counselors, and pharmacists also spend many years preparing to be licensed healthcare providers. In order to increase the penetration of behavioral health services to the many who need them, clinics will need to identify opportunities for people with less training to aid with the delivery. Increasingly, clinics are hiring physician assistants and nurse practitioners instead of the hard-to-fine primary care physician. Similarly, there is increasing use of *Behavioral Health Clinician- Assistants* (BHC-As) to extend the services of BHCs in primary care. BHC-As are capable of providing some assessments and some clinical interventions with BHC supervision (for details, see Chap. 3 in *Behavioral Consultation and Primary Care: A Guide to Integrating Services*). A pilot study conducted by the United States Air Force found that addition of BHC-A services were well received by patients and that their addition increased the penetration of BHC services into the primary care population (Landoll, Nielsen, Waggoner, & Najera, 2018).

4. *Improve access to behavioral health services by changing workflows*: There is tremendous benefit in changing to workflows that improve access to behavior change services. An example is that of the *warm hand-off* suggested by the PCBH model. A warm hand-off occurs when a patient sees a BHC on the same day as their medical visit. The PCC introduces the patient to the BHC, and the BHC sees the patient as soon as possible on the same day. When PCCs are able to introduce BHC services as "short, practical, and immediately available", most

patients readily agree to behavioral healthcare. Another example of a workflow change involves a change in nursing roles. Often, nurses provide triage services to patients phoning in with a request for a same-day visit with the PCC. If allowed to triage patients to a BHC instead of the PCC, nurses may place a variety of patients in same-day BHC appointments, saving PCC appointments for more urgent medical concerns. For example, patients with acute grief, depression, anxiety, and a concern about a child's problematic behavior may be better served in a BHC visit than in a PCC visit. It is desirable to create more complex workflows to better meet the behavioral health needs of complex patients, such as those seeking Medication Assisted Treatment (for examples of more complex workflows, see Robinson & Reiter, 2016, Chap. 12).

5. *Pursue payment reform*: Current payment strategies do not adequately incentivize providers to deliver behavioral health services or patients to seek out behavioral health services. Instead, payment strategies may encourage PCCs to pursue additional testing rather than to delivery less costly behavioral health interventions. Further, current payment strategies promote patient requests for treatment of medical symptoms rather than patient requests for help with being a better mother or father or an effective employee. Payment for healthcare providers do not encourage physicians and behavioral health clinicians to pursue careers in primary care but instead to work as specialists. Those seeking to improve delivery of behavioral health services in primary care need to work diligently with professional groups, state government officials, researchers, and healthcare business planners to re-design incentives. It is possible to recruit physicians into primary care and primary care physicians into rural areas, where the workforce shortage is greatest, by reimbursing their work at competitive rates. It is also possible to influence patient engagement with behavior change services by making these services available and including them as a part of routine good healthcare.

6. *Improve behavioral science training*: Several strategies for improving behavioral science training may be useful in increasing current and future delivery of behavioral health services in primary care. First, both undergraduate and graduate programs need to revamp their curriculum with this aim in mind. More masters level programs designed to prepare students in behavioral health programs are needed. Additionally, fields such as psychology need to develop programs that prepare graduates of a bachelor's program to work in a primary care context. Psychology is the fourth most popular undergraduate degree, yet most people with a psychology degree do not continue in the field. Medical and nursing schools and primary care residency training programs also need to re-shape their curriculum to better prepare physician assistants, nurse practitioners, and primary care physicians for the huge numbers of patients with behavioral health needs that they will serve, day in and day out. Likewise, university departments preparing *Physical Therapists* (PTs), *Pharmacists* (Ph), *Dieticians* (Dt), and exercise specialists need to include training in the basics of brief behavior change early in the course of study. Ideally, universities will support development of inter-disciplinary courses on behavioral health and, in this way, provide an opportunity for the healthcare providers of tomorrow to work in inter-disciplinary teams in undergraduate as well as graduate classes.

Additionally, primary care management can improve clinician access to training on behavioral health by requiring staff to pursue a minimal amount of training. Management can also sponsor brief training during lunch hours or before work. Other possible venues for promoting training are through offering web-based training, ranging from single webinars to on-going coaching. Finally, managers can sponsor adoption of behaviorally-focused care plans by having them included in *Electronic Health Records* (EHRs).

7. *Promote a biopsychosocial approach*: The biomedical model has slowed the delivery of wholistic care to patients of all socioeconomic levels and cultural backgrounds but has perhaps had the most harmful impact on patients challenged by adverse events of childhood. These patients have lived through childhoods rampant with adversity (parental divorce, death or alcohol/drug abuse; sexual or physical abuse; witness of interpersonal violence, etc.). Their on-going exposure to multiple stresses leaves them vulnerable to problematic physical, mental and social health problems. In providing biopsychosocial care beginning at the 2-week well-child visit, we have a better opportunity to break the cycle of adversity and build resilience by identifying and building upon family strengths for surviving—and even thriving.

8. *Focus on patient functioning*: What do you think patients feel when we ask them about symptoms of depression? Many feel embarrassed and ashamed and under-report their symptoms. Why? Everybody wants to be healthy and, at some level, most feel it is somehow their fault if they are not healthy—physically and mentally and especially mentally. Asking patients about their values and their ability to behave in ways that are consistent with their values is much more engaging than asking them if they have been feeling bad about themselves or if they think they are a failure. There is a difference between asking a patient if a person if they are messing up their life and asking a person if they would like to learn new skills to improve the quality of their life. Patients are more likely to engage with healthcare providers when we offer to help them live the meaningful lives they desire and deserve.

9. *Pay attention to resilience*: Up to a third of PCCs report significant symptoms of stress and around a quarter of other members of the PC team report similar problems. This, of course, is a result of the unworkability of current strategies for delivering primary care. When problems occur at such a high rate, it is imperative that clinics begin immediately to monitor stress and to develop on-going programs to address sources of stress and enhance skills for resilience. Resilience is about staying connected to the values that lead a person to pursue a career in healthcare, acknowledging one's self for daily accomplishments, connecting meaningfully with teammates and students of healthcare, and finding a balance between work and the rest of life. There are programs available for use by students and providers of healthcare (for example, see Robinson, Gould & Strosahl, 2010, Chaps. 10 and 11 of *Real Behavior Change in Primary Care: Improving Outcomes and Increasing Job Satisfaction*), and clinics need to build use of these into clinic training days. It is resilience and commitment that provide the fuel for primary care team members to deliver high quality behavior change support to patients.

Table 1.1 Checklist: Recommended strategies for improving delivery of behavioral health services in primary care[a]

Selected strategy	Recommended strategies
	1. Build a team
	2. Use team-based metrics
	3. Use assistants and extenders more
	4. Improve access to behavioral health services by changing workflows
	5. Pursue payment reform
	6. Make training on behavioral science available
	7. Promote a biopsychosocial approach
	8. Focus on patient functioning
	9. Pay attention to resilience

[a]Place a mark beside strategies that you believe would be helpful in your clinic and feasible at this point in time.

Summary

This chapter introduced readers to PC, its mission, and its challenges. The Quadruple Aim provides a benchmark for healthcare quality improvements. The PCMH model provides strategies for improving delivery of primary care services, and the PCBH model describes strategies for bringing behavioral health services into the heart of primary care. Not all clinics will be able to recruit a BHC to work in a fully integrated capacity. However, all clinics can improve their efforts to address the behavioral health needs of patients. To develop a plan for improving behavioral healthcare in their community, we suggest that readers complete the Checklist of Strategies for Improving Delivery of Behavioral Health Services in Primary Care (see Table 1.1). Select the strategies that you think are both feasible and high impact and then find a group of like-minded people to support you in your work. Begin with members of your clinic leadership team; share the Tips for Leaders with them (Table 1.2).

Review of Strategies

1. The inclusion of delivery of behavior health services in primary care will enhance health outcomes.
2. Patient centered medical home and primary care behavioral health are models that describe strategies for improving healthcare outcomes.
3. Primary care faces many challenges to improving delivery of behavioral health services as a part of routine delivery of good healthcare.
4. Readers can start today to improve delivery of primary care behavioral health services in their communities by completing the Checklist of Recommended Strategies for Improving Delivery of Behavioral Health Services and sharing the Tips for Leaders (Table 1.2) with your clinic leaders.

Table 1.2 Tips for leaders

1. Start with your goal in mind – how many patients at your clinic need support with behavior change. Consider the what and how questions (#3 and #4).
2. Form an advisory group and be sure to include one or more patients that would be / are users of behavioral health support services. Share information from this chapter with the group. Modify your goal (#1) so that it aligns with the vision of the advisory group.
3. What and who are your current resources for providing behavior change services to patients?
4. How will you provide training to the staff that provide behavior change services to patients? On-line, on-site? When? How much?
5. Look for funding from non-government organizations and governmental organizations to start additional behavioral services.
6. Find community partners, particularly those who provide behavior change services (or want to start or want to enhance current services). These may include schools, daycare centers, hospital staff, community mental health and substance abuse treatment centers, emergency departments and urgent care centers. Find ways to align your efforts and create consistency in your behavior change methods.

References

Agency for Healthcare Research and Quality. (2014). Defining the PCMH. http://www.pcmh.ahrq. gov. Accessed 14 June 2014. 30.

American Psychological Association Practice Association. (2009). Health care reform: Congress should ensure that psychologists' services are key in primary care initiatives. www.apapractice. org. Accessed 10 July 2013.

Berwick, D. M., Nolan, T. W., & Whittington, J. (2008). The triple aim: Care, health and cost. *Health Affairs, 27*(3), 759–769.

Bodenheimer, T., & Sinsky, C. (2014). From triple to quadruple aim: Care of the patients requires care of the provider. *Annals of Family Medicine, 12*(6), 573–576. https://doi.org/10.1370/afm.1713

Freeman, D. (2011). Blending behaviorists into the patient centered health care home. In N. A. Cummings & W. T. O'Donohue (Eds.), *Understanding the behavioral health care crisis: The promise of integrated care and diagnostic reform*. New York, NY: Routledge.

Hoff, T., Weller, W., & DePuccio, M. (2012). The patient-centered medical home: A review of recent research. *Medical Care Research and Review, 69*(6), 619–644.

Hunter, C. L., Funderburk, J. S., Polaha, J., Bauman, D., Goodie, J. L., & Hunter, C. M. (2017). Primary Care Behavioral Health (PCBH) model research: Current state of the science and a call to action. *Journal of Clinical Psychology in Medical Settings*. https://doi.org/10.1007/s10880-017-9512-0

Institute of Medicine (US) Committee on the Future of Primary Care (1996). Primary care: America's health in a new era. Donaldson, M.S., Yordy, K. D., Lohr, K. N., & Vanselow, N.A. (Eds). Washington (DC): National Academies Press (US); 1996. http://www.iom.edu/CMS/3809/27706.aspx. Accessed 23 June 2005.

John, J. R., Ghassempour, S., Girosi, F., & Atlantis, E. (2018). The effectiveness of patient—Centered medical home model versus standard primary care in chronic disease management: Protocol for a systematize review and meta-analysis of randomized and non—randomized controlled trials. *BioMed Central Systematic Reviews, 7*, 215. https://doi.org/10.1186/s13643-018-0887-2

Landoll, R. R. Nielsen, M. K., Waggoner, K. K., & Najera, E. (2018). Innovations in primary care behavioral health: a pilot study across the U.S. Air Force. TBM. Published by Oxford

University Press on behalf of the Society of Behavioral Medicine. https://doi.org/10.1093/tbm/iby046

Peikes, D., Zutshi, A., Genevro, J. L., Parchman, M. L., & Meyers, D. S. (2012). Early evaluations of the medical home: Building on a promising start. *American Journal of Managed Care, 18*(2), 105–116.

Reid, R. J., Coleman, K., Johnson, E. A., Fishman, P. A., Hsu, C., et al. (May 2010). The group health medical home at year two: Cost savings, higher patient satisfaction, and less burnout for providers. *Health Affairs, 29*(5), 835–843. https://doi.org/10.1377/hlthaff.2010.0158.

Reiter, J. T., Dobmeyer, A. C., & Hunter, C. L. (2017). The Primary Care Behavioral Health (PCBH) model: An overview and operational definition. *Journal of Clinical Psychology in Medical Settings, 24*(4). National Committee for Quality Assurance 2011.

Robinson, P. J., Gould, D., & Strosahl, K. D. (2010). *Real behavior change in primary care. Strategies and tools for improving outcomes and increasing job satisfaction.* Oakland, CA: New Harbinger.

Robinson, P. J., Oyemaja, J., Beachy, B., Goodie, J., Bell, J., Sprague, L., Maples, M. & Ward, C. (2018). Creating a primary care workforce: Strategies for leaders, clinicians, and nurses. *Journal of Clinical Psychology in Medical Settings, 20*(3). https://doi.org/10.1007/s10880-017-9530-y

Robinson, P. J., & Reiter, J. D. (2007). *Behavioral consultation and primary care: A guide to integrating services.* New York, NY: Springer.

Robinson, P. J., & Reiter, J. D. (2015). *Behavioral consultation and primary care: A guide to integrating services* (2nd ed.). New York, NY: Springer.

Rosenthal, T. C. (2008). The medical home: Growing evidence to support a new approach to primary care. *Journal of the American Board of Family Medicine, 21*(5), 427–440.

Siefel, M., & Nolan, K. (2012). *A guide to measuring the triple aim: Population health, experience of care, and per capita cost.* IHI Innovation Series white paper. Cambridge, MA: Institute for Healthcare Improvement. http://www.IHI.org. Accessed 6 June 2014.

Starfield, B. (2008). Refocusing the system. *New England Journal of Medicine, 359*, 2087–2091.

Starfield, B., Shi, L., & Macinko, Q. (2005). Contribution of primary care to health systems and health. *The Millbank Quarterly: A Multidisplinary Journal of Population Health and Health Policy, 83*(3), 457–502.

Chapter 2
Team Work in Primary Care

Abbreviations

ACT	Acceptance and Commitment Therapy
AHRQ	Agency for Healthcare Research and Quality
ARNP	Advanced Registered Nurse Practitioner
BHC	Behavioral Health Clinician
BHC-A	Behavioral Health Clinician-Assistant
BSN	Bachelors Science in Nursing
CBT	Cognitive Behavioral Therapy
CEO	Chief Executive Officer
CHES	Certified Health Education Specialist
CHW	Community health worker
CL	Clinic leaders
COO	Chief Operation Office
DO	Doctor of Osteopathy
ED	Emergency Department
EHR	Electronic Health Record
HC	Health Coach
LPN	Licensed Practical Nurse
LP	Liaison Psychiatrist (or psychiatric prescriber)
MA	Medical Assistant
MAT	Medication Assisted Treatment
MBI-HSS (MP)	Maslach Burnout Inventory-Human Services Survey for Medical Personnel
MD	Medical Doctor
NA	Nursing Assistant
ND	Naturopathic Doctor
PA	Physician Assistant
PC	Primary Care
PCC	Primary Care Clinician
Ph	Pharmacist
PT	Physical Therapist
PT-A	Physical Therapist Assistant

P. J. Robinson, *Basics of Behavior Change in Primary Care*, SpringerBriefs in Psychology, https://doi.org/10.1007/978-3-030-32050-8_2

PCBH   Primary Care Behavioral Health
PCMH   Patient Centered Medical Home
RN   Registered Nurse

We can improve delivery of behavioral health services by working well together in teams and continually identifying and refining strategies for assisting patients with skills needed to address problems of living and pursue vitality. When health care providers work in inter-professional teams, patients are more able to access the expertise they need to work with challenges to their health. A team approach also supports continuity of care, increasing the likelihood that patients will hear similar messages of support and encouragement from all members of the team. While these advantages have the potential for positive impact on patient engagement and clinical outcomes, day-to-day delivery of team-based care can become challenging for individual members of the team and for the team itself. When team members lack skills for promoting cooperation and/or connections with supportive clinic leaders, individual job satisfaction and connection to the team's mission weaken and the team may struggle with pursuing its mission.

Elinor Ostrom, an American political economist, won the Nobel Prize for her work on understanding how groups of people work together to make optimal use of common resources, such as forests, pastures or irrigation systems. In many ways, primary care (PC) services are a common resource for people and the many, many teams of people who provide it may benefit from understanding Ostrom's core *pro-social* design principles. By applying these principles to team operations, teams may become more cooperative and effective and this in turn supports worker satisfaction and allegiance. In this chapter, readers learn about core team members of a behaviorally enhanced primary care clinic and prosocial principles they may use to enhance their work. We also suggest strategies for assessing and addressing burnout, as it is a common problem in primary care at this point in time.

The Team and Their Work

Clinic size and location influence the design of a primary care team and the ways the team attempts to deliver improved behavioral health services to patients. For example, urban areas tend to have more professional staff available for primary care work than rural areas do. Teams in small clinics tend to be made up of standard primary care providers and they may need to enrich their team's expertise through telehealth relationships with externally located healthcare professionals. Whatever the size or location of a primary care team, the work of individual team members tends to change on an on-going basis to some extent, with loss or addition of staff members and shifting responsibilities.

In this section, we introduce team members that are typically present in primary care. We define their roles and describe their training. Then, we introduce newer primary care behavioral health team members. To accomplish a goal of enhanced delivery of behavioral health services, clinics need to link with these professionals to benefit from their more extensive training in behavioral science. These professionals may be fully integrated into the team or working externally in another primary care clinic or in a secondary mental health service. We will suggest additional *external* healthcare staff needed to augment PC team services. Of course, urban, suburban and rural clinics will differ in team membership and efforts to deliver better behavioral health services. We illustrate possibilities with several examples. Before we begin the introductions, let's take a look at how PC is organized.

The Organization of Primary Care

A primary care clinic, depending on its size, may have one primary care team or many. Whether the team has many members or a few, its work is to serve the preventive, acute, and chronic care needs of a defined population of patients (their *panel* of patients). Many of the patients on a primary care panel remain on their panel throughout the lifespan. Panel size varies from clinic to clinic and is smaller for Primary Care Clinicians (PCCs) that provide care for more complex patients, e.g., patients with HIV or patients enrolled in a street youth clinic.

The size of a panel is also adjusted according to availability of teammates to assist with delivery of services. One estimate is that a primary care team can provide reasonable care for a panel size ranging from 1387 to 1947 patients (Altschuler, Margollus, Bodenheimer, & Grumbach, 2014). Their estimates for a panel size of 1387 assumed that teammates would cover 50% of preventive care activities and 25% of chronic care activities. Their estimate for a panel size of 1947 assumed more assistance from teammates (i.e., coverage of 77% of preventive care and 47% of chronic care). Whatever the panel size and the constellation of team members serving them, the health of the team members and the team itself are fundamentally important to their effectiveness in delivering care.

Internal Primary Care Staff

Most primary care clinics involve services delivered by one or more PCCs, a mix of nursing staff, and a variety of staff that provide operational support. Staff members may be part- or full-time. The most recently arriving primary care staff include Behavioral Health Clinicians (BHCs, also called Behavioral Health Consultants) and their assistant counterpart, Behavioral Health Clinician-Assistants (BHC-As). Some clinics also have Health Coaches (HCs) and Community Health Workers (CHWs) on their teams. Clinical pharmacists (Ph) are also pursing integrated work in PC.

Primary Care Clinician

In this book, the term Primary Care Clinician (PCC) includes physicians as well as nurse practitioners (ARNPs), physician assistants (PAs), naturopathic physicians, and any other provider who independently oversees all aspects of a patient's care. In this definition, dieticians, BHCs, acupuncturists and some others may be "clinicians," in the sense that they provide care, but they are not PCCs because they do not govern all aspects of care. The PCC works as a generalist, in contrast to clinicians who work as specialists. As a generalist, the PCC provides care for any undiagnosed sign, symptom or health concern for a patient of any age, the origin of the problem (biological, psychological, or social) or the organ system involved. The PCC is the first point of contact for care and assumes responsibility for on-going care, in consultation with other health professionals as needed. The PCC is also responsible for coordinating a patient's use of additional health care resources to address healthcare needs.

PCP Training

The term physician applies to *doctors of medicine* (MD) and osteopathy (DO). Primary care physicians have training in one or more PC specialties, including family medicine, general internal medicine, geriatrics, and general pediatrics. Some PC physicians obtain additional certification for practicing obstetrics-gynecology. Primary care physicians represent slightly less than one-third of practicing physicians in the U.S. (Agency for Healthcare Research and Quality, AHRQ, 2014).

The Institute of Medicine of the National Academies (1996) recommends the following competencies for PC physicians:

- Periodic assessment of asymptomatic patients
- Screening and early detection of disease
- Evaluation and management of acute illness
- Evaluation and management (or referral) of patients with more complex problems
- Ongoing management of patients with chronic disease
- Coordination of care among specialists
- Provision of acute hospital and long-term care services

Of note, available research suggests that when PC physicians do use behavioral strategies, they tend toward use of cognitive behavioral therapy (CBT) interventions for treatment of depressed patients (Robinson et al., 1995). Also, the likelihood that a PC physician will use behavioral interventions may increase over time when a behavioral health clinician (BHC) works in the clinic (Katon et al., 1996). Historically, residency training for PC physicians in behavior change strategies has been limited. Every family medicine residency program must have a "behavioral scientist" on faculty, usually a psychologist or social worker. However, training usually focuses on didactics regarding diagnosing and psychotherapy interventions, observation of the behavioral scientist in 55-minute family therapy interventions, and home visits with the behavioral scientist. Much of this does not apply to the real world of 15-minute visits in PC.

However, innovation is occurring in some family practice residency training programs, and results suggest improvement in the preparedness of physicians to deliver behavioral health services. In the Central Washington Family Medicine residency program, BHCs are clinician faculty members, and residents work side-by-side with them during rotations in psychosocial medicine. The residents observe multiple brief BHC visits with patients and, when ready, provide parts of the BHC visit and then the entire visit (with direct BHC supervision). Eventually, residents function autonomously as BHCs, providing brief behavioral health visits and consulting with the BHC preceptor only when needed. At CWFM, residents also participate in group medical visits with the BHC. Many other residency programs are also attempting to improve how they prepare the PC physicians to deliver behaviorally focused interventions as a routine part of medical care. Like mental health providers who have tried providing traditional therapy co-located in PC, traditional behavioral scientists working in family practice residency training clinics are realizing that the behavioral health services needed in PC are significantly different from those learned for traditional therapy.

Non-physician Primary Care Clinicians

Non-physician PCCs are usually Advanced Registered Nurse Practitioners (ARNPs) or Physician Assistants (PAs). ARNPs can diagnose, treat and prescribe without physician involvement in some states. To address the workforce shortage of PCCs and to lower salary costs, many organizations are hiring more ARNPs and PAs. By 2025, the number of ARNPs practicing in PC is expected to nearly double (Auerbach et al., 2013). The number of PAs in PC is also expected to grow (Coplan, Cawley, & Stoehr, 2013). Unlike an ARNP, a PA requires physician supervision. PAs and ARNPs will be important members of Patient Centered Medical Home (PCMH) teams (Cooper, 2007).

ARNP and PA Training

Typical PA training involves 18–24 months of graduate work, following a bachelor's degree. An ARNP is usually a registered nurse (RN) who also holds a master's degree in advanced practice nursing.

Naturopathic Physicians

Some states license naturopathic physicians (NDs) to practice PC medicine; their scope of practice and prescriptive authority varies from state to state. While emphasizing use of natural healing agents in patient care, NDs are trained in pharmacology, and in some states such as Washington, Oregon, California, and Arizona, they are licensed to prescribe most synthetic drugs.

ND Training

NDs complete 4–5 years of post-graduate training in a naturopathic medical school. They study the same basic and clinical sciences as MDs, but also receive considerable training in nutrition, counseling/psychology, and homeopathic and botanical medicine. Additionally, they receive extensive training in physical medicine and can provide manipulation treatments (similar to osteopathic or chiropractic manipulation). ND training emphasizes disease prevention and wellness (American Association of Naturopathic Physicians, 2014).

Registered Nurses

Most clinics will have one RN for every five or six PCCs, and they provide a variety of important services in PC, including chronic disease management (e.g., diabetes education, chronic depression), preventive services (e.g., anticipatory guidance during well child checks), and lifestyle behavior change (e.g., smoking cessation). Some focus on specific patient groups and are called disease management RNs or care managers. Others may have responsibilities related to helping patients avoid unnecessary use of the emergency department (ED) and unnecessary hospitalizations by helping at transition points. RNs may also be responsible for triaging patients who call or come to the clinic requesting same-day appointments. RNs with a bachelor's degree may work in an administrative capacity, providing operational support and supervision for nursing and nursing assistant staff.

RN Training

Nursing staff may have one of several degrees, including a bachelor's degree in nursing or an associate degree in nursing.

Licensed Practical Nurses, Nursing Assistants and Medical Assistants

Licensed practical nurses (LPNs), nursing assistants (NAs) and medical assistants (MAs) play important roles in PC. Health care clinics are hiring more LPNs and NAs to assume some duties that would otherwise be accomplished by a RN, given the on-going shortage of nurses.

Nursing staff work closely together to coordinate a variety of patient care activities, beginning with bringing patients into the exam rooms and completing pre-visit activities. They take vitals, clarify the reason for the visit, and verify medications. Additionally, they may ask screening questions about smoking or other problems prior to the patient seeing a provider. They enter pre-visit information into the EHR for the PCC to review. At the end of the visit with the PCC, the NA or MA escorts the patient to the next stop, such as the laboratory or front desk. They may also complete other after-visit activities, such as providing patients with information about resources and patient education pamphlets, as directed by the PCC. For this reason, the BHC (if the clinic has one) should ensure they have access to handouts on behavioral topics and keep them informed about relevant community resources. In this book, we use the term MA consistently, but recognize that NAs may have similar responsibilities.

LPNs, NAs, and MAs

LPNs, NAs, and MAs have completed specialized coursework following graduation from high school. Of the three, LPNs have the most training; NAs, the least.

Support Staff in Primary Care

Support staff include front desk workers, staff who answer the phones and schedule appointments, and staff responsible for billing activities. Depending upon the size of the clinic, one person may be charged with all of these tasks. In larger clinics, multiple staff are needed to complete the work of supporting delivery of PC services.

Front Desk Staff Members

The job of the front desk staff member is to greet the patient, obtain necessary information and generate documentation for the visit. If EHRs are in use, they enter data to indicate that the patient has arrived. If not, the front desk staff member will notify the MA in person about patient arrival. At the end of a visit, patients may turn in a billing slip, pay and/or schedule a follow-up appointment with the front desk staff member. In addition to providing services to patients with scheduled appointments, the front desk worker may also enter same-day patients into PCC and nurse schedules. Front desk staff members have a difficult job and may benefit from learning about how unmet behavioral health needs may play a role in how some patients present for care.

Ward Clerks

Ward clerks provide a variety of services, such as creating provider schedules and making changes to them, scheduling appointments, and facilitating patient referrals.

Appointment Line

In larger clinics, there may be one or more appointment line workers. They answer the phone and assist patients with scheduling appointments.

Billing Specialists

Billing and coding staff record and process patient health records. They organize patient files and assure that visit notes are accurate and accessible. Additionally, they may send out bills and process insurance claims.

Interpreters

Clinics vary in the way they address their needs for interpreting. A small practice may rely on phone interpretation services. Federally qualified health centers, which see a disproportionately large number of non-English speakers, are required as a condition of funding to provide interpreter services. In places like Hawaii, where patients speak 10–15 different languages, clinics tend to have multiple interpreters on staff. Clinics where many patients speak the same non-English language (usually Spanish in the U.S.) tend to hire staff members that are fluent in that language. For patients who speak less-common languages, interpreters from outside agencies may be scheduled for on-site or phone interpretation of a patient's visit.

Administrators

There are a variety of administrators in PC, including medical directors, nursing directors, clinic managers, and Chief Executive Officers.

Medical Directors

A PCC usually fills the role of medical director; their job is to assure that PCCs have team member support for their panel size and the complexity of their patients. They manage PCC staff, support implementation of clinical policies and practices (e.g., diabetes care guidelines), and participant in quality improvement activities (e.g., assisting teams with meeting quality metrics).

Nursing Director

Small clinics may have one RN, but larger clinics or those that are part of a larger organization often have more, including a director of nursing. The director supervises RNs with responsibilities for various departments in a healthcare system and has responsibility for addressing difficulties charge nurses may have related to their supervision of RNs and other nursing staff.

Clinic Manager or Director

The clinic manager may have medical or business training, or both. They are responsible for all aspects of clinic operations. They oversee the budget, purchase supplies, manage the clinic property, and complete personnel work. The manager often supervises reception, billing, and maintenance staff. Managers also work closely with clinical leadership.

Other Leaders

In larger systems with multiple clinics, there may be a Chief Executive Officer (CEO) and a Chief Operating Officer (COO). The Chief Executive Officer (CEO) may work with a senior management team and a board. The CEO is responsible for stating the vision for the organization and defining the strategies to pursue that vision. The CEO also works on budgets and develops and sustains community partnerships.

The Chief Operating Officer (COO) makes decisions about production and work policies. They review statistics about numerous operations within the clinic(s) and monitor quality, safety and efficiency. Using this information, they work with others on policy changes. Overall, the goal of the COO is to optimize the quality of health-care services, assure financial viability for the clinic or system and support attainment of high customer satisfaction ratings.

Primary Care Behavioral Health Team Members

In a behaviorally enhanced primary care team, there will be a variety of new team members, and, in this section, we describe these members who will support team efforts to deliver high impact behavioral health services to patients they see and to patients they do not see face-to-face, but influence by way of educating team members and preparing patient education materials. These include the Behavioral Health Clinician (BHC), the Behavioral Health Clinician-Assistant (BHC-A), the Health Coach (HC), and the Community Health Worker (CHW).

Behavioral Health Clinician

The Behavioral Health Clinician (BHC) is a provider with an independent license to practice in a health care setting. The BHC may hold a PhD/PsyD in psychology, a master's degree in social work, or a master's in counseling or marriage and family counseling. In some countries, such as New Zealand, mental health nurses work in the role of BHC. BHCs work in the primary care clinic as a fully integrated members of the team, providing patient care and support to PCCs and nursing staff (e.g., reviewing records, drafting letters, making calls to coordinate care). Clinical services include delivery of brief, consultation-based visits to patients. At minimum, BHC schedules allow for up to 14 patients visits in an 8-hour day and strive for high patient volume. The schedule template has 30-minute units, with every other visit reserved for same-day patient appointments. Approximately half of a BHC's visits each day are with same-day patients and the remainder may be with scheduled patients. The ratio of same-day to future scheduled slots may vary, depending on the maturity of a BHC practice. At start-up, a BHC may have more same-day slots and then taper these as the practice develops.

BHCs are responsible for helping the team provide preventive, acute, and chronic care services and attain quality metrics. Like PCCs, the BHC sees patients of all ages. Any patient with a problem that has a behavioral component is a good referral for the BHC (ranging from medication adherence, to reducing blood pressure, to improving marital satisfaction). BHCs see individuals and families and provide follow-up in a consultative structure. This means they follow-up, along with the PCP, until the patient has started to improve and has a clear plan in place for continued improvement. At that point, the BHC stops planned follow-up but can always be re-engaged in the case of new or recurring problems.

BHCs are generalists and work collaboratively with healthcare team members in the clinic and in the community to create new workflows that improve outcomes. BHCs use evidence-based behavioral interventions for both psychological and biological problems and teach interventions to teammates over time. Some BHCs assist with coordinating care for patients seen in the emergency department (ED) or hospital. In an effort to improve outcomes to patients with greater risk for poor health, BHCs work with team members in piloting and then implementing pathways designed to involve the BHC consistently in delivering evidence-based interventions to members of the targeted group (e.g., patients with chronic pain). Robinson and Reiter (2015) provide guidance on developing pathway and group services. Some but not all pathways involve group medical visits. BHCs provide other group-based services, such as workshops and class series, often co-leading groups with a teammate.

Larger healthcare systems are beginning to create two levels of BHCs. A level one BHC provides clinical services, while a level two BHC has additional responsibilities. These additional responsibilities include training, supervision, program development, research and publication, and management. Since it would be impossible for a level 2 BHC to provide full-time clinical services and complete all of these additional tasks, a level 2 BHC typically reduces hours devoted to providing clinical services when taking on leadership roles such as clinical training and supervision, program development, program evaluation, and management responsibilities. It is best for level 2 BHCs to continue with some clinical services, as they have higher levels of competence and provide a model of excellence for new BHCs. Additionally, their connection with "front line" work empowers them to innovate within the service and evolve its impact. There are many opportunities to adjust the workload of level two BHCs to match their unique interests and abilities. It is important to mention minimal requirements for a level two BHCs include having practiced as a BHC for 6–12 months, demonstrated expected metrics (e.g., productivity; fidelity to the PCBH model by maintaining a 1:1 ratio of same-day to scheduled visits and 1:2–3 ratio of initial to follow-up visits; high satisfaction ratings from PCCs, RNs and patients), and started one or more pathways and groups supporting behavior change.

BHCs complete graduate courses of study and become licensed by their states. Most behavioral health providers need additional training to work successfully in the Primary Care Behavioral Health (PCBH) model. This training typically occurs in three phases. The initial training involves classroom study of the PCBH model and conceptualization, assessment, and intervention materials detailed in Chaps. 3, 4, and 5 of this book. Trainees also practice skills from these chapters in skill practice exercises in Phase one in order to prepare for Phase two training. For phase two, a BHC trainer shadows the new BHC in their home clinic and assists them with developing the skills they need for adequate demonstration of BHC competencies. The BHC trainer uses the BHC Competency Tool (see Robinson & Reiter, 2015, Chap. 5) to evaluate the performance of the new BHC after 2–3 days of shadowing and coaching the BHC as they deliver services to patients and interact with their new team members. The BHC trainer also provides some brief training in the PCBH model to all staff during the 2–3 day Phase two period. Phase three continues for a 6-month period when BHC trainers continue to be available in live webinars, where new BHCs can learn more clinical skills and problem solve barriers to optimal integration in their clinics.

Behavioral Health Clinician Assistant

The Behavioral Health Clinician Assistant (BHC-A) provides services to extend the impact of the BHC in a clinic, working closely to support the overall needs of the PC team. BHC-As increase the productivity of a BHC by completing portions of the visit such as greeting the patient in the waiting room and completing pre-visit activities, such as introducing the BHC service to patients referred for an initial visit and completing the BHC outcome visit measure. For same-day referrals to the BHC, the BHC-A may enter the patient on the BHC schedule and start the BHC chart note. BHC-As may be bilingual and bi-cultural and, in addition to providing interpretation services, they may assist by providing short behavioral health skill practices with patients when the BHC does not speak the native language of the patient. BHC-As also assist the BHC in delivery of group-based services, escorting patients to the group room, starting chart notes, and completing billing slips. BHC-As also monitor behavior change handouts used by the BHC, nurses, and PCCs and re-stock them when needed. Finally, BHC-As may monitor registries of select patient groups and make brief calls to patients to support implementation of behavior change plans.

Often, BHC-As are medical assistants who have long-term experience in the clinic and sought out training from the BHC to prepare for BHC-A work. Because they are also able to provide MA services, they can provide those services when an MA is out of clinic if the BHC is able to manage their practice without support.

Health Coach

Health coaches (HCs) use specific clinical interventions, including motivational interviewing, to engage patients in health behavior change. Their work often focuses on patients who have chronic conditions and those who face multiple barriers to use of healthcare, including language barriers and a lack of experience with healthcare providers. The health coach role is similar to the BHC-A role but differs in a few ways. First, HCs have typically completed trainings that prepare them to deliver evidence-based behavior change interventions for specific problems, such as tobacco use or problematic lifestyle behaviors. They can easily assume the tasks of a BHC-A but may need support in learning teamwork skills, as this may not have been provided in the brief trainings they receive in health coaching. The original health coach role encouraged community-based work with patients that were not engaged with primary care. The goal was to encourage the patient to engage with PC services. Like BHC-As, HCs are often bi-lingual and bi-cultural and work well with patients who share their language and culture. They may see patients for individual and group visits, and they often work with patients by phone.

Health coaches complete a certificate training focused on skills for engaging patients in conversations about health and promoting health behavior change. While some HCs may have a bachelor's degree in Health Education, the training of others consists of on-the-job training or completion of a certificate programs after high school graduation. HCs participate with BHCs and BHC-As (in clinics with BHC-A) in Phase one PCBH training activities.

Community Health Worker

Community health workers (CHWs) may be members of the team that focus on improving care to patients that have a specific disease (e.g., HIV/AIDS) or on patient groups (e.g., pregnant women or children). They may be responsible for population-based care initiatives in the clinic (e.g., improving nutrition or promoting immunization). For PC clinics serving higher risk patients (such as public health department clinics), CHWs provide essential services for engaging patients in care and changing health behaviors.

CHWs typically have at least a high school diploma and have completed a brief period of on-the-job training. Some states have certification programs for community health workers, and some clinics may require the Certified Health Education Specialist credential for CHWs. CHWs may be graduates of certificate programs or hold a bachelor's degree, or even a master's in social work. They are skilled at engaging patients and tend to have strong skills for understanding cultural and racial factors related to health-care engagement. Health educators need a bachelor's degree.

Other Possible Primary Care Behavioral Health Team Members

As PC teams expand, there will be defined roles and responsibilities for additional behavioral health clinicians. Some will be located in primary care and others will be located externally. These include Clinical Pharmacists, Addiction Medicine Physicians, and Psychiatric Prescribers. The success of interventions initiated by Physical Therapists (PTs) and Physical Therapist Assistants (PT-As) might be enhanced by their becoming closely connected with primary care behavioral health team members. Integration of PT services is needed, given the large number of patients with pain-related conditions, including those with pain related to chronic diseases and injuries.

Internal location of pharmacists, PTs, and PT-As would also promote better continuity of care and increased opportunities to enhance outcomes by close coordination with integrated behavioral health staff. Some health care systems are using the strategies of the PCBH approach to create fully integrated roles for professionals traditionally located externally, such as pharmacists (see Gallimore, Corso, Robinson & Runyan, 2018). While well received by PC team members, there are barriers to widespread integration efforts, including the exclusion of payment for pharmacist services by most federal and private payors. However, over time, payment reform will hopefully shift to encourage integration to achieve added value.

Behavioral health specialists located externally and serving the PC team in liaison roles will likely increase, particularly with advancements in tele-health services. Inclusion of a *liaison psychiatrist* (LP) as an externally located team member is more feasible with recently released collaborative care codes. The services of externally located addiction medicine specialists will also be very helpful to primary care clinics, particularly those who offer *Medication Assisted Treatment* (MAT) Recovery programs for patients with opioid use disorder. MAT Recovery, by definition, involves medication treatment with counseling or behavioral interventions. It is possible that PCCs will feel more confident in prescribing naltrexone and buprenorphine when BHCs are routinely involved with MAT patients and addiction medicine specialists are available for consultation. Additionally, MAT patients may be more likely to sustain MAT participation if BHCs are available to address common co-morbidities (such as chronic pain, depression, and post-traumatic stress disorder). BHCs often play key roles in facilitating communication between the members of the internal team and external team members working in liaison roles and providing consultation services as needed.

A Note about Teamwork in Urban, Suburban, and Rural Clinics

Urban and suburban clinics are usually larger than rural clinics and the size of a clinic will determine the size of the team (and the number of teams), as well as the variety of disciplines represented on the team(s). Larger clinics that are part of a larger healthcare system may be more able to recruit staff for evolving towards a behaviorally enhanced PC team, particularly in suburban and urban areas where more behavioral health and medical professionals are available. Diversity of professional team members facilitates patient access to a broad range of services and strong coordination of care. To obtain this diversity in rural areas, clinics may need to offer higher salaries or alternatively to pursue it through technology. Small clinics can enhance their expertise through tele-health relationships with externally located team members, including BHCs and LPs.

Team organization and use of communication strategies is also influenced by proximity of a clinic to external healthcare resources. The PC team in a *frontier* clinic may be that of a single PA, a MA, and one support staff. In First Nation communities, the PC staff may be a single MA and a BHC-A who are tribal members living in a small village a plane-ride away from PC clinic-based services. For more remote clinics, the relationship between the local and remote staff needs to support delivery of preventive, acute and chronic care services. Regular contact and planning, as well as service at the time of request, provide a foundation for the development of strong relationships between local and remote staff.

A rural clinic in Idaho's efforts to improve delivery of behavioral health services offers a good example of what is possible, even with limited resources. The clinic team included a part-time ARNP, a part-time PA, and a full-time support staff member that provided front desk, phone, scheduling, and billing support. To promote increased delivery of behavioral health services, the team began using a package of 1-page, evidenced-based patient education handouts for common health concerns (e.g., sleep problems, using specific positive praise with children, letting go of anger, becoming active, learning to relax, etc.). The front desk worker created a registry that allowed her to track patients who were given a handout and to call them and check on its usefulness. This small internal team developed a relationship with an externally located BHC in their region. The BHC offered consultation and case reviews as needed and developed behavioral health education materials as requested. Additionally, the BHC provided regular live webinars on behavior change topics.

Enhancing delivery of behavioral health services in a larger system with more resources might look very different. For example, the system might integrate changes to the electronic health record (EHR) to support consistency of PCC, nursing, and BHC staff in using a care plan supporting behavior change for a specific group, such as patients experiencing difficulties with achieving control over diabetes (see for example, the Bull's-Eye in Chap. 5 of this book). A BHC-A might provide phone calls to patients after clinic visits to support implementation of behavior change experiments planned in BHC visits. Additionally, BHCs might work with other members of the behaviorally enhanced team, such as integrated PT-As or dieticians, in providing group medical visits to patients with diabetes (or other difficult problems, such as chronic pain). Whether rural, suburban, or urban, the quality of team relationships and a can-do attitude fuel creativity in pursuing improvements in delivery of behavioral health services to patients.

Prosocial Teams

Teams vary in the quality of their relationships and the processes they use to guide the work they do; some have better relationships and are highly cooperative, while others struggle and have frequent turn-over in team membership. A more cooperative team is more successful in meeting the healthcare needs of patients on their panel. In this section, we suggest some group design principles for teams to use to promote team health and better success in implementing behavior change programs. These ideas are from the Prosocial Project, a project developed to support greater levels of cooperation in groups. The prosocial movement originated from the work of Elinor Ostrom, a political scientist whose lifelong work resulted in identification of specific principles describing how groups that obtain the best outcomes for use of common resources operate (Hayes, accessed 6-12-2019). We review eight of these principles and provide ideas about how they might apply to the work of a primary care team attempting to address the medical and psychological needs of patients on their panel.

1. *Group boundaries are clearly defined.* For primary care teams, this principle points to the importance of clearly defining their goal for improving behavioral health for their patients. This would require them to understand behavioral risk factors for members on their panel. For example, a panel with a large group of older adults might anticipate that many patients would experience some level of de-moralization with the challenges of aging and that they would benefit from group medical visits that included delivery of behavioral health services to strengthen their skills for healthy aging and to lessen the social isolation that can occur in later decades of life. The team would embrace a common direction of supporting healthy aging and plan accordingly as to what they could and would do to support this direction.

2. *Rules for governing use of common goods match the local needs and conditions.* This principle suggests that the team is responsible for on-going exploration of ways to use the resources of the team to achieve an optimal health outcome for all of the patients on their panel. So, the team might be faced with prioritizing possible initiatives to promote better behavioral health. Often, many programs are possible and team members may vary in interests leading to a lack of consensus. Dr. Ostrom's principle emphasizes the importance of including all team members in a process that leads to consensus about the work of the team. For example, a BHC on a team might want to check-in with all patients who come for well-child visits. However, there may be inadequate resources for the BHC to participate in all well-child visits and to also provide group medical service visits for an identified group of 50 patients over age 75 with multiple medical conditions. A rule or guide adopted by the team might be that of using the BHC to achieve optimal penetration into the patient panel on any given day, such that they might not provide well child visit support on days when multiple group medical visits for the older patients are planned.

3. *Those affected by the rule can participate in modifying the rules.* In other words, patients, clinic leaders, all members of the team, and support staff serving multiple teams need to participate in creating and modifying rules pertaining to the work of the team.

4. *Outside authorities respect the right of team members to make the rules for the team.* This principle concerns the fundamental importance of the team believing that they have the authority to make important decisions about how they complete their work. Pro-social teams would see the clinic manager as a resource for helping them perform operations needed to improve delivery of behavioral health services.

5. *The team develops a system for completing its work; the community supports implementation, and there is on-going monitoring of individual member behavior.* This principle concerns the primary importance of a close working relationship between patients on the panel and the team providing their care. Whether the system is addressing needs for preventive care or acute care, a pro-social strategy would be to enlist community support. Involving patients in the work of the team may take different forms. The team might conduct a survey in order to understand patient perspectives on behavioral health issues. Alternatively, the team might convene a focus group to learn more about patient opinions and ideas. For specific behavior change programs, a team would be wise to form an implementation committee that includes patients from the panel, particularly those that would be impacted by the program.

   This principle also alludes to the need to have a method of obtaining data about team and patient behaviors of key importance to any system developed by the team. Metrics would include the extent to which patients engaged in the program's services, the level of satisfaction associated with services received, and whether the services should continue. Developing a plan to evaluate programs encourages cooperation and risk-taking by team members and patients. Optimally, team members feel free to "think outside the box" in planning for the behavioral health needs of their patients. When they do, they can learn a lot from program attempts that fail and progress more rapidly toward success. Data allow teams to fail quickly and mindfully.

6. *Use graduated sanctions for rule violators, beginning with mild sanctions and increasing incrementally.* This design principle applies to team members as well as patients in the panel. For teams to implement workflows well, all members need to perform tasks associated with their role consistently. Sometimes individuals are drawn away from team agreements by needs to excel and be recognized for their individual accomplishments. Other times, a team member's ability to function optimally in an agreed upon workflow is a result of their being distracted by negative thoughts and feelings toward another team member. Sanctions need to include efforts to understand the context for the rule violation and to identify any skills the team member may need in order to better comply with workflows or other team agreements.

   An example of applying this design principle to patients is that of a team plan to address patient use of urgent or emergent care services for routine health problems. An initial sanction might be that of a team member calling the patient to explore their choice to use a higher level of care than needed and to clarify their understanding about the benefits of using primary care for non-urgent healthcare problems. With repeat violations, sanctions might build toward visiting the patient's home and/or requesting that patient meet with multiple members of the team to discuss ways the team can care for the patient and their family, consistent with actual resources available for addressing healthcare needs for all patients on the panel. The patient would be offered a range of options consistent with resources, such as receiving regularly scheduled phone visits to trouble-shoot psychosocial and medical problems and availability of access to same-day primary care clinic visits with the member of the team member requested by the patient.

7. *Provide accessible, low-cost means for dispute resolution.* This principle might apply to the team's efforts to address the requests for care by patients with health anxiety, such that patients might be offered a brief meeting with a PCC and BHC to discuss behavioral health strategies for addressing life stress and working with worry, particularly worries about the challenging problem of undiagnosed or poorly understood symptoms.

8. *Build responsibility for governing the common resource in nested tiers from the lowest level up to the entire interconnected system.* The lowest tier in the context of a primary care clinic is that of an individual inter-professional team and their panel of patients. Support and management staff associated with the team are also a part of the fundamental group that then connects with other teams and with the larger healthcare system. A team's responsibility would include developing workflows that coordinate delivery of highly satisfying services to their patients and for connecting patients with resources at higher levels of care external to the primary care clinic. All levels would be responsible for monitoring the outcomes of their work and for making changes that improve the operation of the larger system.

These principles are food for thought for primary care providers, whatever their role, as they support a view of health as a common resource important to all members of a community. Ideally, teams will review these design principles and use them to stimulate their thinking about ways to cooperate for the common good inherent in promoting better behavioral health. An on-going process of discussion, decision-making and assessment creates a context for creativity and experimentation; both are important to the goals of cultivating healthy teams and promoting better behavior health in the patients they serve.

Acceptance and Commitment Therapy

Acceptance and Commitment Therapy (ACT) is an approach initially tested with clinical patient samples that is now known to be of benefit to the health of managers and workers in a variety of work settings (Flaxman & Bond, 2006). A version of ACT known as ACT at Work defines strategies for optimizing the psychological flexibility of a group or organization (Flaxman, Bond, & Livheim, 2013). ACT promotes psychological flexibility by encouraging people to focus on the present moment and, depending upon the opportunities available, to take action toward achieving their goals and values, even when experiencing difficult or unwanted thoughts and feelings (Hayes, Luoma, Bond, Masuda & Lillis, 2006). Psychological flexibility is important in the work context and in the clinical context of patient care. Chapters 3, 4, and 5 provide information on using ACT and Focused Acceptance and Commitment Therapy (FACT) (i.e., ACT adapted for brief intervention settings) in Chaps. 3, 4, and 5.

Higher levels of psychological flexibility in the workplace are associated with a greater sense of well-being for workers and with greater success in work activities (Flaxman, Bond, & Livheim, 2013). Let's take an example to illustrate how psychological flexibility impacts the work of a group. Let's imagine that a team member feels frustrated or angry in response to something said by another member of the team. If unable to let go of these difficult thoughts and feelings, the teammate may begin to feel discouraged and fail to engage in actions needed to support the work of the team in the moment. ACT at work interventions focus on helping team members learn skills for detecting difficult thoughts and feelings, as they are an inevitable part of working together, and to allow them to be there rather than adding to them by trying to ignore them or by justifying them. While difficult, team members can learn to accept difficult thoughts and feelings with compassion and to view them as just a part of "the human condition" rather than their only reality. Then, they are more able to quickly re-direct their attention and effort to the task at hand.

ACT at work trainings also assist team members with clarifying their individual values and identifying values shared by the team. With on-going skill practice and planning, team members come to support each other. They are more able to anticipate difficult moments, where unpleasant thoughts and feelings are likely to come up and make it more difficult for the team to succeed. Examples of stressful moments that teams may be able to anticipate and plan for include being short-staffed, working with an angry blaming patient or responding to a patient's suicide. In anticipating the difficult thoughts and feelings that are likely to come up in these situations, teams may be able to pre-plan and practice small exercises that help members step back from unhelpful judgements and evaluations and respond instead with greater compassion, both for themselves and for patients.

While space does not allow us to provide further details about the ACT at work curriculum here, we encourage readers to explore Dr. Bond's work and the ACT at Work Matrix and to use it to promote psychological flexibility at individual and team levels. Dr. Bond's book, *The Mindful and Effective Employee*, provides a curriculum for enhancing psychological flexibility in the work context (Flaxman, Bond, & Livheim, 2013), and, if there is a BHC on your team, perhaps they will be able to follow Dr. Bond's curriculum and provide the class for your team, including your clinic leaders.

A Word About Resilience

Teams that know how to cooperate and that have healthy connections with externally located resources tend to be healthy teams and to create a work environment that promotes resilience. However, some team members will still experience high levels of stress and become vulnerable to what has been referred to as *burnout*. Burnout is a state of exhaustion resulting from difficulties in coping with overwhelming, long-term stress and resulting in a dwindling interest in work.

Christina Maslach and colleagues (Maslach, Schaufeli, & Leiter, 2001) described three main components of burnout: emotional exhaustion, depersonalization, and a lack of personal accomplishment. Emotional exhaustion is feeling emotionally drained and depleted in response to excessive psychological demands. Depersonalization involves a person's efforts to distance themselves from their emotional responses, which results weaker connections with team members as well as patients. A third feature of the burn-out experience is the person's diminishing sense of personal accomplishment.

The Maslach Burnout Inventory

There are a number of surveys available for assessing burn-out. An ideal option is the Maslach Burnout Inventory-Human Services Survey for Medical Personnel (MBI-HSS (MP) (available on line from Maslach and Jackson). The MBI-HSS (MP) is a variation of earlier surveys developed by Maslach and her team, and it is adapted for medical personnel (Maslach & Jackson, 2018). The most significant alteration in this version is a change of "recipients" to "patients". The 22-item survey is self-administered, and team members may elect to use it annually as a check-up or on an as needed basis.

Because burnout is a dynamic interaction between a person and their work context, teammates may notice signs of burnout in a teammate before the teammate does. When a teammate moves closer to a state of burnout, teammates see the team member as more distant from the teammates, less emotionally responsive, "just going through the motions of work" and less likely to participate in planning and evaluating the team's work. With an understanding of burnout, teammates are less likely to be frustrated and to respond in unhelpful ways to the struggling member and, instead, to be more skillful in reaching out and offering a helping hand. A team that understands burnout and believes that every member's mental health is important to the team may be more able to honestly and openly encourage team members to take time to care for themselves and address problems outside of work. A team that is informed about burnout is more able to suggest that a colleague seek care from an Employee Assistance Program and to check on the teammate's progress over time.

Compassion-An Antidote for Stress

Given the fast-pace and high stakes of primary care work, it may difficult for team members to slow down, relax and feel the connections with others that are important in all helping activities. Taken literally, compassion means "to suffer together." Emotion researchers define compassion as the feeling that arises when one perceives another's suffering and experiences a desire to relieve it. Compassion differs from empathy and altruism in that it involves the desire to help. Brain scientists are beginning to map the biological basis of compassion, and with more information we can better understand the evolutionary purpose of compassion. When one feels compassion, their heart rate slows, and regions of the brain linked to empathy, care-giving, and feelings of pleasure become active. It is the activation of the compassion process that stimulates our efforts to help others. The following three exercises are examples of protocols that a team might use to light up the compassion areas of their brains. Many others are possible and reading these may prove useful to the team in evolving their own practices.

Morning Huddle Compassion

This exercise brings a moment of compassion to the morning team huddle. As a part of reviewing the list of patients scheduled for the day, one or more team members may voice a connection with a particular patient and a desire to help. In response, the team can take a minute in silence to respect that desire, each member working to activate a sense of caring for that patient. Any team member can identify any patient, and there is no need to create a detailed plan for helping, although there may be standard procedures or practices planned. This small practice focuses on bring-ing openness to seeing new ways to help a patient that is struggling.

End of Day Gratitude Circle

This exercise encourages team members to recognize moments of gratitude for the work of individual team members and the team itself. It is simple and straight-forward and can be a practice at the end of the day where the team comes together for 5 minutes of reflection. During this exercise, each team member makes a state-ment of gratitude. Statements may be directed toward a personal experience with a patient, an observation of the work of a teammate with a patient, or the efforts of a teammate to help another teammate. Teammates who leave before the end of the day may leave a written statement to be read by a teammate during the gratitude circle.

Self-Compassion

For many people, it is easier to feel compassion for others than to feel compassion for one's self. Given this tendency, it is important for the team to practice an exer-cise that promotes feelings of compassion toward the self. As a part of morning or afternoon huddling, the team might observe a few moments in silence to set an intention of compassion in their work. Examples of intentions include: "May you feel safe. May you feel calm. May you smile a lot today. May find moments to slow down. May you forgive quickly. May you express gratitude. May you show yourself kindness." Members may formulate their own unique intention. This list of possibilities could be placed on a team bulletin board and serve as a reminder to practice self-compassion.

Recommended Strategies for Promoting Healthy PC Teams

The important goal of developing strong primary care teams requires on-going attention by PC team members and support from administrative and operational staff. To encourage a systematic approach to this goal, we offer a checklist of recommended strategies (see Table 2.1 Checklist: Recommended Strategies for Developing Healthy Teams Capable of Helping Patients with Behavior Change). Individual strategies are more appealing to different teams at different times, so readers are encouraged to select the one or two that will provide the best impetus for creativity, effectiveness and resilience in your clinic at this time.

1. *Evaluate current staff resources and potential for increased delivery of behavior health services.* What does your staff know how to do and have interest in doing to improve the behavioral health of patients on their panel? Are there patient education pamphlets on common behavioral health problems in the clinic? What is the evidence base for these pamphlets? Who has time and expertise to offer brief behavior change support in the clinic? If you have a BHC, are they trained in the PCBH model or working in a traditional role where they provide hour-long visits to a small number of patients over extended periods of time? This approach results in most patients with behavioral health needs receiving little or no support at all, and it can be changed. Chapters 3, 4, and 5 provide information on assessment and intervention strategies that will allow the team to reach more patients. Whatever your resources, it is best to pursue a population-based care approach to behavioral health change where a *little* support and skill training is provided *for a lot* of people.

2. *Form a plan to increase your team's resources for delivery of behavioral health services.* What additional resource is most feasible for your team at this point in time? Is there funding to support training in behavioral health assessment and intervention for a single or multiple members of a team? Often, training one team member is a great start, particularly if they are encouraged to "teach the skills forward" to the team over time. Is there funding for initiating an on-going consultation relationship with an externally located behavioral health professional? If so, we recommend that you pursue consultation with a BHC that is trained in PCBH competencies and in the contextual behavioral science methods described in Chaps. 3, 4 and 5 in this book (for more information, see Robinson & Reiter, 2015, Chap. 5 for a description of PCBH competencies for BHCs).

These practical methods are easy for PC team members to learn, and they work for patients with psychological *and* medical problems. Is there funding for adding a BHC to your team? If so, plan carefully about how to recruit and hire someone who will work well in this new role for behavioral health providers. Guidance for writing a job description, posting an advertisement, conducting interviews, and selecting an employee are available (See Robinson & Reiter, 2015, Chap. 3 for detailed information). Given the newness of the BHC role, most good candidates will need additional training and mentoring, so budget for this and make a plan before hiring.

3. *Encourage teams to consider prosocial design principles and learn to be more psychologically flexible.* Do team members perceive their team to be working well together? Are they satisfied with their jobs? Do they feel that they can make changes to improve the quality of their working relationships and the outcomes of their work? Ideally, answers to all of these questions will be affirmative. In reality, they may not be. Asking the questions is a first step. Introduce the idea of improving the team's ability to focus on team outcomes and of finding ways to increase compassion and cooperation skills. A brief discussion of prosocial design may be useful, and someone in the clinic may be interested in reading Dr. Bond's book, *The Mindful and Effective Employee* (Flaxman, Bond, & Livheim, 2013).

4. *Assess and address stress and stress overload; plan for resilience. Healthy teams happen in contexts that support health at work.* An integral part of health at work programs is identifying the sources of stress and making needed changes, whether to the workplace, the team's workflows or skills, or the individual staff member's need for restoration from stress overload. Stress overload (or burnout) is an all too common problem for healthcare staff. Do your teams routinely assess stress levels and sources of stress? Is there a process for checking on symptoms of stress overload? If not, start a discussion and planning process at your clinic. A variety of materials are available to assist your work (see Robinson, Gould, & Strosahl, 2010, Chaps. 10 and 11 for information on assessing stress and starting a resilience program).

5. *Encourage daily routines that promote kindness and self-compassion.* Do your teams have morning huddles or an end-of-the-day routine? Building these into the schedule can set the stage for better planning and evaluation of workflows on a daily basis and create opportunities for growing the practice of kindness toward others and self that can easily buffer the stress of providing high stakes services at a fast pace. This chapter offers several routines for teams, but members of your team may have ideas of their own.

6. *Strengthen connections with community.* Take stock of resources in your community that deliver services related to behavioral health. Does your team have a good relationship with them? How could you strengthen these relationships? Health fairs may promote a spirit of collaboration in a playful context, and they may facilitate opportunities for co-training and combined efforts to address the

health needs in the community, such as safe, clean parks. Regular lunch and learn activities for team members and community healthcare providers also provide opportunities for building relationships.

7. *Initiate programmatic efforts to address behavioral health needs.* Do your teams have a current program that targets care to a specific group of patients on the panel? If not, this strategy might help build the team's self-efficacy for making a difference. Many programs are possible, and they may target prevention or patients living with chronic conditions. For example, a clinic might initiate a pilot program with a prevention focus by developing a brief workshop for families with children between 10 and 14 years of age that informs them about vaping and the marketing campaign that vaping companies use to target children and teenagers. The team could invite staff from local schools and/or share resource materials with the schools in their area to extend the impact of their efforts. Another example is that of a program to improve engagement in care by patients living with multiple chronic health conditions. The program could feature a monthly or quarterly family event on Saturdays. Patients could come with their families to a potluck featuring healthy local foods. Topics of discussion could include family values concerning health and family relationships, having fun with meal preparation, and great topics for conversation at meal time. Programmatic efforts heighten a team's sense of purpose and offer opportunities for creativity. They provide team members with a reason to learn new skills and to experiment with working in new roles. All of these factors may contribute to better job satisfaction and retention of team members.

Table 2.1 Checklist: Recommended strategies for developing healthy teams capable of helping patients with behavior change

Selected strategy	Recommended strategies
	1. Evaluate current staff resources and potential for increased delivery of behavior health services.
	2. Form a plan to increase your team's resources for delivery of behavioral health services.
	3. Encourage teams to consider prosocial design principles and learn to be more psychologically flexible.
	4. Assess and address stress and burnout; plan for resilience.
	5. Encourage daily routines that promote kindness and self-compassion.
	6. Strengthen connections with community.
	7. Initiate programmatic efforts to address behavioral health needs.

[a]Place a mark beside strategies that you believe would be helpful in your clinic and feasible at this point in time.

Summary

In this chapter, readers met the traditional members of PC and the newly arriving team members of advanced inter-professional PC teams. The chapter provided examples of innovations spawned by the group design principles discovered by Elinor Ostrom. Additionally, the chapter introduced the work of Dr. Frank Bond on psychological flexibility and health at work. Resilience programs and intentional practice of small exercises to promote kindness, cooperation and self-compassion may promote better team health, particularly in today's PC clinics where stress overload is common. The Checklist of Recommended Strategies for Developing Healthy Teams Capable of Helping Patients with Behavior Change (See Table 2.1) can help readers select targets that are feasible and high impact. With targets for improving team health and a group of like-minded people to support your work, change for the better will happen. Be sure to discuss your ideas with your leadership group and let them know about the Tips for Leaders at the end of this chapter (see Table 2.2).

Review of Strategies

1. Traditional PC staff include PCPs, nursing staff, administrative staff, and a variety of support staff members.
2. BHCs and BHC-As are new and well received PC team members. They offer consultative services to patients, nursing staff, and PCPs. They provide preventive, acute and chronic care services to patients of any age.
3. External BH team members working in a liaison capacity include prescribers of psychotropic medications for psychiatric problems and addiction medicine specialists offering support to PC Medication Assisted Treatment Recovery programs.
4. Teams need to use the resources available to them to enhance behavioral health services. Smaller and more remotely located teams need agreements with regional tele-health services that include BHCs and LPs.
5. Teams may benefit from discussing Elinor Ostom's design principles for groups. It is imperative that the limited resource of healthcare be used well and this relies on the work of highly cooperative groups working together at different tiers of healthcare.
6. Acceptance and Commitment Therapy (ACT) at Work is an educational program that teaches strategies to PC managers and teams. In less than 5 hours of class instruction, workers can become more psychologically flexible and perform their jobs with greater resilience.
7. There are ways to assess for symptoms of stress overload and burnout, and ongoing assessment allows teams to better detect warning signs and to intervene early.

8. Small exercises in a team's daily routines may increase kindness at work and promote connection to the many inspiring moments that happen every day in caring for patients.
9. A variety of strategies may be useful in developing strong PC teams, capable of delivering powerful behavioral change services to patients. Use the Checklist in Table 2.1 to select the strategies that may prove useful at this time. Ask your clinic leadership to take a look at the Tips for Leaders in Table 2.1, as their support is important to your success.

Table 2.2 Tips for leaders

1. Support development of telehealth capacity and provide telehealth training for staff.
2. Promote ways of working that promote cooperation. Listen and learn from team ideas stimulated by review of the design principles.
3. Encourage innovation in development of behavioral health services. Support meaningful evaluation and encourage the process of fail fast, fail often, and fail mindfully.
4. Facilitate reports on behavioral health processes and outcomes from electronic health record data (e.g., number of patients with chronic disease with at least one BHC visit, health related quality of life scores for adults aged 65 and older). Provide colorful charts that show status and targets for each PC team.
5. Obtain ACT at work training for teams, from your clinic BHC, a regional BHC, or an organizational psychologist. Measure job satisfaction, team productivity, and patient satisfaction before and after the training.
6. Encourage on-going evaluation of stress and pursue strategies for addressing factors in the work context. Work with an Employee Assistance Program (EAP) that offers evidence-based care for stress overload and burnout. Assure that staff know of the quality of the EAP service and the evidence for the services they offer.
7. Encourage teams to develop their own daily routines for promoting compassion and good will.

References

Agency for Healthcare Research and Quality (AHRQ). (2014). Defining the PCMH. http://www.pcmh.ahrq.gov. Accessed 4 June 2014.

Altschuler, J., Margollus, D., Bodenheimer, T., & Grumbach, K. (2014). Estimating a reasonable patient panel size for primary care physicians with team-based task delegation. *Annals of Family Medicine, 10*(5), 396–400. https://doi.org/10.1370/afm.14007

American Association of Naturopathic Physicians. (2014). Accessed at http://www.naturopathic.org. Accessed 20 Aug 2014.

Auerbach, D. I., Chen, P. G., Friedberg, G. W., Reid, R. O., Lau, C., et al. (2013). Nurse-managed health centers and patient-centered medical homes could mitigate expected primary care physician shortage. *Health Affairs, 32*(11), 1933–1941.

Cooper, R. A. (2007). New directions for nurse practitioners and physician assistants in an era of physician shortages. *Academic Medicine, 82*(9), 827–828.

Coplan, B., Cawley, J., & Stoehr, J. (2013). Physician assistants in primary care: Trends and characteristics. *Annals of Family Medicine, 11*(1), 75–79.

Flaxman, P. E., & Bond, F. W. (2006). Acceptance and commitment therapy in the workplace. *Mindfulness-Based Treatment Approaches*. https://doi.org/10.1016/B978-012088519-0/50018-6

Flaxman, P. E., Bond, F. W., & Livheim, F. (2013). *The mindful and effective employee: An acceptance and commitment therapy training manual for improving well-being and performance.* Oakland, CA: New Harbinger.

Gallimore, C., Corso, K. A., Robinson, P. J., & Runyan, C. N. (2018). Pharmacists in primary care: Lessons learned from integrated behavioral health. *Medical Practice Management*, 321–325.

Hayes, S. C. ACT and the core design principles. https://www.prosocial.world/post/act-and-the-core-design-principles. Accessed 6 Dec 2019.

Hayes, S. C., Luoma, J. B., Bond, F. W., Masuda, A., & Lillis, J. (2006). Acceptance and commitment therapy: Model, processes and outcomes. *Behavior Research and Therapy, 44*(1), 1–25.

Institute of Medicine of the National Academies. (1996, January 01). Primary care: America's health in a new era. Washington, DC: Institute of Medicine. http://www.iom.edu/CMS/3809/27706.aspx. Accessed 23 June 2005.

Katon, W., Robinson, P., Von Korff, M., Lin, E., Bush, T., et al. (1996). A multifaceted intervention to improve treatment of depression in primary care. *Archives of General Psychiatry, 53*, 924–932.

Maslach, C., & Jackson, S. (2018). The Maslach Burnout Inventory – Human Services Survey for Medical Personnel (MBI-HSS (MP). Available on line: https://www.mindgarden.com/mbi-human-services-survey-medical-personnel/698-mbihssmp-individual-report.html.

Maslach, C., Schaufell, W. B., & Leiter, M. P. (2001). Job burnout. *Annual Review of Psychology, 52*, 397–422. https://doi.org/10.1146/annurev.psych.52.1.397

Robinson, P., Bush, T., Von Korff, M., Katon, W., Lin, E., et al. (1995). Primary care physician use of cognitive behavioral techniques with depressed patients. *Journal of Family Practice, 40*(4), 352–357.

Robinson, P. J., Gould, D., & Strosahl, K. D. (2010). *Real behavior change in primary care. Strategies and tools for improving outcomes and increasing job satisfaction.* Oakland, CA: New Harbinger.

Robinson, P. J., & Reiter, J. D. (2015). *Behavioral consultation and primary care: A guide to integrating services* (2nd ed.). New York, NY: Springer.

Chapter 3
Behavior Change in Primary Care: The Basics

Abbreviations

AAQ-II   Acceptance and Action Questionnaire-II
ACT   Acceptance and Commitment Therapy
BHC   Behavioral Health Clinician
CBT   Cognitive Behavioral Therapy
FACT   Focused Acceptance and Commitment Therapy
PC   Primary Care
PCC   Primary Care Clinician
PF   Psychological Flexibility
SDOH   Social Determinants of Health

It is easy to look at a plant in a garden and see that it is flourishing … or that it is not. A plant that is failing to flourish may have a weak central stem. It may have no new shoots and may be dropping its flowers. Its leaf stalks may be drooping, and its leaves fading from their healthy natural color. It is much the same for people in their communities who are failing to flourish; their loss of vitality is visible. Sadly, communities often struggle with tending to people whose life conditions are not promoting their engagement in meaningful lives. Fortunately, primary care is an institution where detection of problems with thriving is easy, and even better, the *Primary Care* (PC) team is there to proactively promote flourishing from birth to the end of life.

This is the perspective on behavior change described in this chapter: the goal of behavioral health services in PC is to help people flourish. This is accomplished by identifying and addressing barriers to flourishing. Is the plant in a location that doesn't support thriving? If so, can it be moved, and, if not, what changes to are possible to help it thrive, even without a change in location? Are there soil amendments, a change in watering, a stake to support it that will encourage the plant back to its natural state of vitality? This chapter introduces new, evidence-based methods for promoting health in patients who need help in returning to their natural state of seeking health and growth.

© The Author(s), under exclusive license to Springer Nature
Switzerland AG Pte Ltd 2019
P. J. Robinson, *Basics of Behavior Change in Primary Care*, SpringerBriefs
in Psychology, https://doi.org/10.1007/978-3-030-32050-8_3

Signs of failure to flourish in humans, as in plants, offer important clues as to what intervention and change has the greatest potential for helping. An effective behavioral science for primary care offers PCCs, BHCs, nursing staff, and other PC staff tools for exploring, identifying and intervening. A functional approach to assessment seeks to identify contextual factors and to inform development of powerful interventions for behavior change. This chapter introduces these tools and concludes with recommendation of five specific strategies for readers to use in cultivating a new perspective on the what, how, and why of behavior change. These strategies provide the basics of behavior change in primary care, and, of the five, understanding the function of a problem behavior, is particularly challenging.

What Do Patients Want?

While most people want to flourish, research suggests that many are not. In fact, one study of European countries reported rates of flourishing ranging from a low of 6% in the Russian Federation to a high of almost 35% in Denmark (Huppert & So, 2009). Keyes & Haidt suggested a rate of 40% for Americans (Keyes & Haidt, 2013). Before looking at what blocks flourishing, let's define flourishing and attempt to understand its relationship to commonly experienced mental problems. Martin Seligman originally proposed use of the term, flourishing, to describe the process of finding fulfillment in life, accomplishing worthwhile tasks, and connecting meaningfully with others— "the good life" (Seligman, 2012). Professor Lynn Soots added to the definition of flourishing, describing it as experiences of inner happiness occurring in the context of pursuing one's values, riding the peaks and valleys of life, and experiencing a sense of accomplishment (Soots, 2018).

Flourishing and mental and biological problems are probably best thought of as occurring on different dimensions, as one can have a mental problem or a biological disease and still experience flourishing. A group of researchers in the Netherlands examined the impact of flourishing on development of recurrent mental disorders over a 3-year period (Schotanus-Dijkstra, ten Have, Lamers, de Graaf, & Bohlmeijer, 2017). In this large study of 4482 adults, the flourishing measure categorized patients into low and high flourishing groups-based on well-being scores (life-satisfaction, happiness) and eudemonic well-being scores (social contribution, purpose in life, personal growth). Results suggested that flourishing reduced the risk of incidence of mood disorders by 28% and of anxiety disorders by 53% but did not significantly predict substance use disorders. The patterns of association were the same for either high hedonic or high eudemonic well-being. Significant results were found for substance use disorders when life-events and social support were removed as covariates.

Flourishing may provide some protection against development of mental problems and improve our ability to bounce back from physical illness and injury. Developing skills that support development of a nurturing support group appear to buffer the impact of stress. When PC teams promote flourishing, they may reduce the rates of patients progressing toward development of disease, promote rapid recovery from illness or injury and better support self-management among patients with chronic disease.

So, flourishing is not the absence of mental or biological illness; it is the ability to live well even in unfavorable conditions, including difficult biological, psychological and social conditions. Of course, negative conditions do impact flourishing; however, they need not stop it. Flourishing ebbs and flows in one's life, in response to life circumstances, and it is often a person's ability to access health care services that make all the difference in skills they use to address on-going problems of living.

Measurement of Flourishing

There are a variety of scales available for measuring flourishing. The Flourishing Measure was developed by the Human Flourishing Program, and it was first described in a 2017 paper presented by Professor VanderWeele in the Proceedings of the National Academy of Sciences (VanderWeele, 2017). The Human Flourishing Project encourages tracking of flourishing in medical, workplace, educational, and government settings. The measure is copyrighted under a Creative Commons License and can be used without permission for non-commercial purposes if proper citation is given (See reference list: VanderWeele, 2017).

The original flourish measure consisted of two questions from each of five domains: happiness and life satisfaction, mental and physical health, meaning and purpose, character and virtue, and close social relationships. A more recent version includes financial and material stability as a sixth domain. Questions for the scale were selected primarily from well-being measures with empirical validation. Respondents use a scale of 0–10 for each question. The sum of the first five domains provides a "flourishing score" (range: 0, not flourishing whatsoever to 100, highest possible flourishing). Including the sixth domain in the sum results in a "secure flourishing score" (range: 0–120). See Table 3.1 for a copy of the flourish measure.

The Flourishing Measure provides a quick read on a person's level of flourishing and can help clinicians begin a conversation about challenging circumstances in life and one's need to grow and to experience a sense of wellness during these times. The secure flourishing score may be particularly useful when there are concerns about a patient's finances or access to basic resources. Another strategy for using this measure is to obtain scores from all patients on an annual clinic "Flourishing Day". Results would provide a population health estimate of flourishing in the clinic. This measure could be assessed year to year to evaluate the impact of clinic-wide efforts to promote higher levels of flourishing.

Table 3.1 The flourishing project measure[a]

Domain	Questions	Score
Happiness and life satisfaction	1. Overall, how satisfied are you with your life as a whole these days? 0 = Not satisfied at all, 10 = Completely satisfied 2. In general, how happy or unhappy do you usually feel? 0 = Extremely unhappy, 10 = Extremely happy	
Mental and physical health	3. In general, how would you rate your physical health? 0 = Poor, 10 = Excellent 4. How would you rate your overall mental health? 0 = Poor, 10 = Excellent	
Meaning and purpose	5. Overall, to what extent do you feel the things you do in your life are worthwhile? 0 = Not at all worthwhile, 10 = Completely worthwhile 6. I understand my purpose in life. 0 = Strongly disagree, 10 = Strongly agree	
Character and virtue	7. I always act to promote good in all circumstances, even in difficult and challenging situations. 0 = Not true, 10 = Completely true of me 8. I am always able to give up some happiness now for greater happiness later. 0 = Not true of me, 10 = Completely true of me	
Close social relationships	9. I am content with my friendships and relationships. 0 = Strongly disagree, 10 = Strongly agree 10. My relationships are as satisfying as I would want them to be. 0 = Strongly disagree, 10 = Strongly agree	
Financial and material stability	11. How often do you worry about being able to meet normal monthly living expenses? 0 = Worry all of the time, 10 = Do not ever worry 12. How often do you worry about safety, food, or housing? 0 = Worry all of the time, 10 = do not ever worry	

[a]VanderWeele, T.J. (2017). On the promotion of human flourishing. Proceedings of the National Academy of Sciences, U.S.A., 31:8148–8156.

Barriers to Flourishing

Social Determinants of Health (SDOH) and the experience of multiple adverse events in childhood may impact a person's likelihood of flourishing. SDOH include where patients live, work, learn and play and the impact of these circumstances on health. Poverty limits a person's access to healthy foods, healthcare, and safe neighborhoods, while education is associated with better health (Maryland Department of Housing and Community Development, 2016; Minnesota Housing Finance Agency, 2016; U.S. Department of Agriculture, 2016). PC team members are wise to recognize and address the impact of social and physical environments on a patient's health and to moderate these to whatever extent possible by connecting patients with community resources. Healthy People 2020 provides guidance on SDOH and identifies a goal of creating social and physical environments that promote good health for all people (United States Department of Health Office, 2019).

The experience of adverse events during childhood is common, with as many as one in three reporting experiences of abuse, neglect, and / or disruption in their households (e.g., divorce, violence, etc.). Adults with a history of multiple adversities have more mental and physical health problems as adults and they are at greater risk for premature mortality (Felitti, Anda, Nordenberg, Williamson, Spitz, et al., 1998). They also have more chronic health conditions and more surgeries.

However, some beat the odds and develop resilience (Poole, Dobson, & Pusch, 2017). Positive attitudes, supportive relationships, and spirituality may moderate the impact of adversity on health (Cesene, 2016) and on flourishing (Keyes, 2009). Keyes (2009) compared flourishing in groups of Black and White people and reported that Blacks demonstrated higher levels of flourishing than Whites and greater resilience to some mental problems. This finding suggests that some moderators may have a powerful influence on highly negative stresses, such as social inequality and long-term exposure to discrimination (Keyes, 2009).

On-going research by a Calgary group of clinicians working in primary care and Professor Keith Dobson suggest that patients with a history of multiple childhood traumas may benefit significantly from brief behavioral health interventions delivered by clinicians in PC. Specifically, participation in a series of six primary care behavioral health classes designed to enhance their resilience resulted in improvement to depression and anxiety scores. Social health and mindfulness scores also improved during this low intensity behavioral health intervention (Dobson et al., 2017).

PC teams are wise to recognize and use the strength of flourishing to promote health. Clinics in communities with higher concentrations of SDOH factors and different racial groups provide rich opportunities for exploring and encouraging flourishing. To take advantage of these opportunities, teams need to understand the community where they work, to recognize flourishing as a strength, to promote work-arounds for patients that address social and physical environmental constraints on health behavior, and to support community initiatives that address SDOH.

Psychological Flexibility and Inflexibility

When patients fail to flourish, develop mental health problems, or struggle in efforts to cope with medical problems, clinicians need to offer powerful interventions for behavior change. *Acceptance and Commitment Therapy* (ACT), a model of *Cognitive Behavioral Therapy* (CBT), aims to promote flourishing, reduce psychopathology, and facilitate flexible responding to challenges of living, including medical problems (Hayes, Strosahl, & Wilson, 2012). *Focused ACT* (FACT) is a CBT with the same goals as ACT but adapted for the brief visit context of primary care. FACT seeks to help patients move from psychologically *inflexible* ways of responding to problem of living to psychologically flexible ways of responding (for more information, see Robinson, Gould & Strosahl, 2010; Strosahl, Robinson & Gustavsson, 2012).

Table 3.2 The Acceptance and Action Questionnaire-II (AAQ-II)

Below you will find a list of statements. Please rate how true each statement is for you by using the scale below to fill in your choice

1	2	3	4	5	6	7
Never true	Very seldom true	Seldom true	Sometimes true	Frequently true	Almost always true	Always true
1. My painful experiences and memories make it difficult for me to live a life that I would value.						
2. I'm afraid of my feelings.						
3. I worry about not being able to control my worries and feelings.						
4. My painful memories prevent me from having a fulfilling life.						
5. Emotions cause problems in my life.						
6. It seems like most people are handling their lives better than I am.						
7. Worries get in the way of my success.						
Total Score						

[a]Bond, Hayes, Baer, Carpenter, Guenole, et al., 2011.

Before providing a measurement strategy and a clinical definition of *Psychological Flexibility* (PF), let's look at an important study that evaluated the impact of ACT on flourishing (Bohlmeijer, Lamers, & Fledderus, 2015). The study involved a post-analysis of an earlier randomized controlled trial of adults with depressive symptomatology who participated in a guided self-help ACT intervention. Results suggested that participants increased between five and 28% in flourishing, and the effects on flourishing were maintained at the three-month follow-up.

Psychological Flexibility and Avoidance

Psychological flexibility, like flourishing, is a multi-dimensional construct and can be measured. The *Acceptance and Action Questionnaire-II* (AAQ-II) is a measure of psychological flexibly (see Table 3.2, Bond, Hayes, Baer, Carpenter, Guenole, et al., 2011). Many studies using the AAQ-II have found that low psychological flexibility is associated with psychological problems and difficulties with functioning, including anxiety, lower quality of life, poorer work performance, difficulties with learning, and long-term disability (Kashdan & Rotterburg, 2010). The AAQ-II measures one-factor of psychological inflexibility: *Experiential Avoidance* (EA). EA is the efforts a person is making to avoid difficult thoughts, feelings, and sensations. The EA score is a sum of the seven items; higher scores indicate greater levels of psychological inflexibility. In talking with patients about their EA scores, clinicians may describe the results in terms of the level of pressure on a person at that point in time and the person's efforts to avoid or resist the pressures.

In conceptualizing barriers to flexible behavior change, the dynamic between approach and avoidance is of central importance. Table 3.3 provides an Approach-Avoidance tool to encourage readers to begin to consider this dynamic in

Table 3.3 The approach-avoidance tool

	Avoid	Approach
Actions	What behaviors does the patient do to get away from difficult thoughts, feelings, sensations, and situations (e.g., distracting behaviors, drugs / alcohol, etc.)?	What behaviors does the patient do that are consistent with what matters and who matters?
Thoughts **Feelings** **Sensations**	What thoughts, feelings, and sensations does the patient use to control, ignore, suppress, or avoid? What unworkable rule(s) is the patient following?	What matters to the patient? Who matters to the patient? What helpful rule is the patient following?

understanding information about a patient's actions (i.e., observable behaviors) and thoughts, feelings and sensations (internally experienced behaviors). A person's actions, thoughts, feelings and sensations are sorted left (i.e., have a function of avoidance) or right (i.e., serve an approach function). For example, a person who complains of depression may report thoughts about being "useless" or "a failure", a sense of heaviness and low energy, and feeling "numb". All of these internal behaviors would go into the avoidance bottom left quadrant. They represent things the patient wants to avoid and tries to ignore or get rid of. The same person might say that he tries to cope by watching a lot of movies, playing video games, and staying up late to avoid worrying about his problems when he goes to bed. All of these "action" behaviors serve an avoidance function, so they would go in the top left quadrant.

This tool helps *Primary Care Clinicians* (PCCs) and *Behavioral Health Clinicians* (BHCs) keep a patient's strengths in mind and use them in conceptualizing ideas for small changes. By obtaining an understanding of what matters to a patient and what they are already doing that reflects their values, the clinician is able to add behaviors into quadrants on the right side of the Approach-Avoidance Tool (Table 3.3). The behavior of asking a PC team member for help is an example of an action with an approach function. An attentive clinician may hear patients say, "Well, I have recovered from depression before and I did it without those pills" and then ask questions that help the patient further state (and connect with) approach-oriented thoughts, such as, "I do have strengths and I care about my health."

Alternatively, a clinician may hear a patient say, "I still call my mother every week to let her know I'm okay" and then clarify a value of showing love and thoughtfulness to their family members and friends. Empowered by conceptualization of the ways approach and avoidance are operating in the patient's life, PC team members may help patients open to avoided thoughts, feelings and sensations (and to see connections between these difficulties and their values), and perhaps feel more compassion for themselves. With more openness to their difficulties, patients may find a stronger connection with their values, see possibilities for more approach-oriented actions, and engage in their lives with greater vitality.

A Clinical Definition of Psychological Flexibility

From a clinical perspective, psychological flexibility (PF) is a person's ability to be fully present, to understand available options for responding to problems, and to pursue a course of action consistent with chosen values. Psychological inflexibility involves not being present in the moment, being unable to perceive current internal and external experiences and, therefore, unable to see new options for responding and for choosing a course of action consistent with values. There are, of course, many shades of grey rather than absolute flexibility and rigidity. Psychological flexibility is dynamic, changing moment to moment in patients and in clinicians as well.

Greater PF enhances the ability to accept and understand emotional pain and difficulties that arise in the normal course of living. While *psychological inflexibility* means spending more time on resisting or suppressing life problems, PF means accepting difficult thoughts and feelings and spending more time and energy pursuing what matters most. Psychological inflexibility blocks learning, and PF promotes learning, variability in behavior, and vigor in life.

People get "stuck" in their life problems because they rely on their thoughts and emotions as guides for their behaviors. Our thoughts and emotions are sometimes helpful, but they are not always useful guides for making long-term choices. Our thoughts and emotions change constantly. Humans cannot hold on to a feeling they like, such as happiness, any more than they can make a feeling they do not like, say for example, sadness, go away. Our values or principles for living are more reliable anchors for decision-making and charting our courses of action, and humans may easily loose site of these guides when challenges to biopsychosocial health are present.

In summary, flourishing is a positive mental health quality that clinicians can assess and encourage. Flourishing may have a moderating effect on the impact that adverse life conditions have on physical, mental, and social health. Psychological flexibility is a group of processes that help us understand how people get stuck in responding to difficulties, using avoidance-oriented behaviors that may provide some temporary relief but at the cost of dimenishing resources for approach-oriented behaviors that promote flourishing. In Chaps. 4 and 5, there is more information about ACT and FACT, including descriptions of the specific processes that contribute to PF.

Basic Methods for Targeting Behavior Change in Primary Care

Behavior change strategies for primary care need to engage patients and fit the requirements of the primary care context. In primary care, the problem of greatest concern for the patient is the target for behavior change. Most patients ultimately are much more concerned about their functioning than symptom elimination. Even the patient that is disabled by chronic pain will admit that the purpose of their life needs to be bigger than being pain-free.

Recall the example of a person struggling with depression used in the previous section. In conversing with a clinician in PC, that person may decide that the problem of greatest concern to them is not "depression", but instead the "lack of enthusiasm to do the work they once loved and difficulties feeling a strong connection with their work team". In later chapters, readers will learn to take the problem a person brings and through a conversation come to a definition that compels behavior change. This is an important method for behavior change as it further engages patients in care.

Patients need new skills to pursue new solutions to the problems that trouble them. Functional assessment methods are ideal for clinicians in PC because they provide a systematic approach to understanding the patient's problem, its context, and its function. Functional assessment methods enable the clinician to develop behavior change plans that target specific factors maintaining problem behaviors. With a functional assessment, clinicians are able to use evidence-based interventions with greater precision and impact. Functional assessment frees us from the more traditional method of diagnosis and application of a treatment matching the diagnosis.

So, what exactly is involved in functional assessment of a problem behavior? The functional assessment approach detailed in Chap. 4 incorporates both indirect assessment (e.g., results of a health-related quality of life survey the patient may complete prior to a visit) and direct functional assessment (e.g., interview questions, rating scales). Chapter 5 offers readers an opportunity to develop skills that support use of functional analysis, where a clinician intentionally changes factors in the environment during the assessment (e.g., changing positions in the room, asking the patient to stand or to speak at a faster or slower pace) and observes the impact of the change on the problem (e.g., the patient's attention, experience of emotion, etc.).

Functional assessment strategies are processes and they require a lot of highly discriminated professional skill. That being said, these are skills that clinicians can master, and they are well worth persistent study. Clinicians experience more success in patient care that includes identifying and attending to the variables that influence the problem behavior. This approach also shows respect to the patient, as patients appreciate a clinician's efforts to understand the why-when-what-how factors before suggesting change strategies. Functional analysis increases treatment precision and efficacy and promotes development of practical plans. Readers will learn to use functional assessment tools in Chap. 4 (i.e., Contextual Interview Questions), and conceptualize patient care from a functional assessment perspective.

Strategies for Promoting A New View of Behavior Change in PC

While there are many barriers to moving toward routine delivery of accessible, engaging, and clinically effective behavioral health services to PC patients, one of fundamental importance is the lack of a strong vision informed by reliable strategies. A strong conceptualization of the patient's difficulties can inspire and direct our efforts. If you've read this far, you probably believe in the power of primary care to create a community where more and more people flourish, pursuing the meaningful lives they desire and deserve. You are probably also enticed by the theory of avoidance and approach that provides a foundation for conceptualization and for helping people who "get stuck" and need help to flourish. Because systems of healthcare are "big ships" and big ships turn slowly, it will take many, many small community-based primary care clinics working together to turn the ship toward a new conceptualization of health, where behavioral health is a priority. Table 3.4 provides a Checklist of Recommended Strategies for Creating a New Perspective on Behavioral Health that engages patients and healthcare staff, and the section below provides information about each strategy. Readers can use the table to identify several strategies that are meaningful and feasible at this time.

1. *Address behavior change when patients present for care.* This strategy involves a coordinated effort to create a clinic environment that says, "Behavioral health is a priority here". Historically, many PC staff thought of behavioral health as a specialty service for a relatively small number of patients. The role of PC was to diagnosis and refer the few patients who needed care from a specialist. Today, it is clear that this has not worked well—over half of the people referred do not make a connection with a specialty mental health or substance abuse provider and fewer than half of that relatively small group engage in care. Today, there is also a better understanding of the interaction between physical, mental and social health, where problems in one area tend to spread to the other areas of life.

   When a patient presents for care, clinicians need to communicate an interest in behavioral health. A poster in the waiting area might announce an upcoming Saturday afternoon event when patients are invited to a potluck picnic to learn about flourishing, complete a flourishing check-up and make a plan to flourish more! Offering such an activity says that positive mental health is important. Another poster or a letter or an electronic communication to patients might notify patients of the availability of same-day behavioral health services to assist with stress, relationship concerns and other common problems of living. The use of this language communicates the view that personal difficulties are normal, and the PC team is prepared to help at the patient's time of need.

   Of course, PC staff will need to change their appointment templates to create same-day appointments for behavioral health visits. A BH same-day appointment could be booked by patients with a new behavioral health concern or by a patient returning for follow-up of a previous or on-going problem. Patients seek care when psychosocial distress is high, and they are less likely to show for care when distress drops. Many more behavioral health services are delivered when behavioral health appointments in PC are highly accessible. With small changes by the team, patients come to rely more on the team for advice, support, and learning new skills when individual and family problems first arise rather than waiting until problems are more extensive.

2. *Promote the idea that good behavioral health involves learning skills needed to flourish.* All too often, patients assume that they should already know how to be happy, form and maintain loving relationships, and solve the many difficult problems that come into their lives. They may feel isolated, believing they are alone in experiencing frustration, sadness, or anger. In reality, life offers continual opportunities for learning by providing problems, including negative thoughts and emotions. Since this is part of the human situation, these difficult inner experiences are not signs of failure but signals of the need to learn new skills.

3. *Talk with patients about what matters and who matters in their lives.* All too often, when people see a PC clinician, they feel it's necessary to talk about a

physical problem or perhaps a diagnosis or medication they learned about from the media. Clinicians that ask about behavioral factors related to physical complaints help patients change their expectations of PC, and patients learn to consider how behavioral factors often relate to physical, psychological, and social health.

Certainly, a patient's values are related to their requests for help, whether for a physical, emotional, or social problem. If the patient did not care about something related to the problem, they would not have spent the time it took to organize and attend a primary care appointment. "Why is finding a new solution to this problem important at this time?" "Tell me who matters in your life right now." These are probes that create a context of caring and importance in an interaction between a PC clinician and a patient, and they are very useful in this new approach to behavioral health in primary care.

4. *Invite patients to complete routine checks of flourishing and identify barriers.* Clinicians may ask patients to complete the flourishing measure provided in Table 3.1 as a part of the annual adult health check-up. This practice would provide an opportunity for the clinician to talk about the importance of positive mental health and their availability to help the patient address barriers to flourishing, as they tend to come up fairly often for most people. A patient could indicate a concern related to a lower rating on one of the 10 items and a clinician working in PC might be able to offer advice about a possible change the patient could try or about a resource that might prove helpful (e.g., resources for basic needs, a class in the community, a book related to the concern, etc.). When patients identify barriers originated from efforts to control or suppress difficult thoughts and feelings, the clinician can normalize this and provide a very brief description of how the mind works. "The mind is helpful with some problems and not so helpful with others." They can talk about the importance of relating to the mind in different ways at different times. Readers will learn more about how to conduct this type of conversation in Chaps. 4 and 5 of this book.

There are other ways for clinicians to address barriers to flourishing, such as bibliotherapy and PC classes. Many patients would benefit from reading a book, such as *Get Out of Your Mind and into your Life* (Hayes & Smith, 2005). Note that there is also a version of this short, readable book for adolescents (Ciarrochi, Hayes, & Bailey, 2012). Other patients would prefer to attend a class that provides training in psychological flexibility (including how the mind works and how humans can learn to work well with their minds). The Life Path Class is a 3–4 visit program that helps patients identify and make small changes and pursue what matters in life (See Strosahl, Robinson & Gustavsson, 2012 for a description of a curriculum; also, manual available on book website: basicsofbehaviorchangeinprimarycare.com). This important strategy supports more consistent detection of behavioral health concerns, an important aspect of this new approach to health.

5. *Understand the function of a behavior.* This chapter introduced the tools of functional analysis and the Approach-Avoidance Tool (Table 3.3). These tools provide useful guides for expanding from a biomedical focus to a biopsychoso-

cial perspective informed by powerful, evidence-based methods for behavior change. If this strategy appeals to you, start using it by looking at your own life and how the approach-avoidance dynamic operates. Experiment by conceptualizing after a visit with a patient and discuss what you are learning about these methods with a colleague. In Chap. 4, readers learn about additional tools that pave the way for developing precise and practical interventions.

Table 3.4 Checklist: Recommended strategies for promoting a new perspective on behavioral health services in primary care[a]

Selected strategy	Recommended strategies
	1. Address behavior change when patients presents for care.
	2. Promote the idea that good behavioral health involves learning skills needed to flourish.
	3. Talk with patients about what matters and who matters in their lives.
	4. Invite patients to complete routine checks of flourishing and identify barriers.
	5. Understand the function of a behavior.

[a]Place a mark beside strategies that you believe would be helpful in your clinic and feasible at this point in time.

Summary

Rates of psychological problems are increasing, and more patients are developing chronic diseases related to unhealthy lifestyle habits. Access to specialty mental health and substance abuse services continues to be problematic and many patients fail to engage in care, even after waiting a long time for care in the specialty sector. A new vision of how to address behavioral health concerns in primary care is necessary. This chapter introduced the concept of flourishing as an indicator of positive mental health and suggested that PC clinicians can promote flourishing. Psychological flexibility is an important construct for understanding why some patients flourish and others get stuck in behavior patterns that limit or worsen their well-being and sense of purpose in life. This chapter offers healthcare clinicians from all disciplines ideas for conceptualizing a strong approach to behavioral health that interprofessional teams can deploy to improve the health of all people. Flourishing and psychological flexibility are applicable at all levels of healthcare service, including the individual patient-clinician interaction, team relationships and team behavioral health initiatives, the culture of the clinic, and the connection of clinics with community-based organizations. We encourage readers to select strategies that are both feasible and high impact from the list of recommended strategies in Table 3.4 and, then, to share them with a group of like-minded people. A good place to start is talking with a clinic leader and sharing the Tips for Leaders with them (Table 3.5).

Review of Strategies

1. Flourishing is the ability to live well, pursuing meaningful goals and close relationship, even with the challenge of mental or biological illness.
2. Patients can complete the Flourishing Project measure in 5 minutes; it can be used as a screener in wellness visits (see Table 3.1).
3. Some adults who experienced more adverse events in childhood may face more barriers to flourishing in adulthood.
4. Psychological flexibility (PF) is the ability to be fully present, to understand available options for responding to problems, and to pursue a course of action consistent with chosen values.
5. The Acceptance and Action Questionnaire-II (Table 3.2) provides a measure of experiential avoidance or the strength of a person's efforts to suppress or avoid difficult thoughts, feelings, and situations.
6. Focused Acceptance and Commitment Therapy (FACT) is a contextual behavioral science approach to behavior change that guides development of interventions to improve PF in brief visits.
7. The Approach-Avoidance Tool (Table 3.3) supports clinician efforts to conceptualize behavior change from a functional perspective and to identify patient strengths related to pursuing greater meaning in life.
8. A functional assessment of patient problems improves the precision and impact of behavior change interventions.
9. Table 3.4 offers readers an opportunity to identify strategies that will be most useful in promoting a new vision for behavioral health in PC. Readers are encouraged to select a few strategies, discuss them with colleagues, and to share the Tips for Leaders in this chapter with their clinic leaders (see Table 3.5).

Table 3.5 Tips for leaders

1. Provide support for new tools for assessing behavioral health needs, such as the Flourishing Project Measure and the Acceptance and Action-II measure. Both are available for public use, provided that their source is sited.
2. Encourage adaptations to the EHR that facilitate on-going attention to behavioral health processes and outcomes, such as including a flourishing score for all patients every 1–2 years.
3. Support clinic initiatives that focus on developing feasible and effective services to identify patients who have experienced multiple adverse events as children and to address them proactively with feasible resources, such as the EmbrACE program for PC (see https://www.eventscribe.com/2018/ABCT/fsPopup.asp?Mode=presInfo&PresentationID=429471).

References

Bohlmeijer, E. T., Lamers, S. M. A., & Fledderus, M. (2015). Flourishing in people with depressive symptomatology increases with acceptance and commitment therapy. Post-hoc analyses of a randomized controlled trial. *Behaviour Research and Therapy, 65*, 101–106. https://doi.org/10.1016/j.brat.2014.12.014

Bond, F. W., Hayes, S. C., Baer, R. A., Carpenter, K. M., Guenole, N., Orcutt, H. K., … Zettle, R. D. (2011). Preliminary psychometric properties of the acceptance and action questionnaire – II: A revised measure of psychological inflexibility and experiential avoidance. *Behavior Therapy, 42*(4), 676–688. https://doi.org/10.1016/j.beth.2011.03.007

Cesene, D. F. (2016). Understanding the moderators of adverse childhood experiences on mature adult satisfaction and adjustment. Doctoral dissertation. Youngstown State University. OhioLINK ETD Center and the Maag Library Circulation Desk. Accessed 20 May 2019.

Ciarrochi, J., Hayes, l., & Bailey, A. (2012). *Get out of your mind and into your life or teens: A guide to living an extraordinary life*. Oakland, CA: New Harbinger.

Dobson, K., Pusch, D, & Klassen, C. (2017). Workshop 2 – Developing a trauma-informed treatment in primary care: The embrACE model for patients with adverse childhood experiences. Association for behavioral and cognitive therapies, 2018.

Felitti, V. J., Anda, R. F., Nordenberg, D., Williamson, D. F., Spitz, A. M., Edwards, V., … Marks, J. S. (1998). Relationship of childhood abuse and household dysfunction to many of the leading causes of death in adults. The Adverse Childhood Experiences (ACE) study. *American Journal of Preventive Medicine, 14*(4), 245–258.

Hayes, S. C., & Smith, S. (2005). *Get out of your mind and into your life: The new acceptance and commitment therapy*. Oakland, CA: New Harbinger.

Hayes, S. C., Strosahl, K. D., & Wilson, K. G. (2012). Acceptance and commitment therapy. In *The process and practice of mindful change* (2nd ed.). New York, NY: Guilford.

Huppert, F. A., & So, T. T. C. (2009). What percentage of people in Europe are flourishing and what characterizes them? Prepared for the OECD/ISQOLS meeting "Measuring subjective well-being: An opportunity for NSOs?", Florence, July 23–24, 2009. http://citeseerx.ist.psu.edu/viewdoc/download?. Accessed 21 June 2019 10.1.1.550.8290&rep=rep1&type=pdf.

Kashdan, T., & Rottenberg, J. (2010). Psychological flexibility as a fundamental aspect of health. *Clinical Psychology Review, 30*(7), 865–878. https://doi.org/10.1016/j.cpr.2010.03.001

Keyes, C. L. (2009). The black-white paradox in health: Flourishing in the face of social inequality and discrimination. *Journal of Personality, 77*(6), 1677–1706. https://doi.org/10.1111/j/1467-6494.2009.00597.x

Keyes, C. L. M., & Haidt, J. (2013). *Flourishing: Positive psychology and the life well lived*. Washington, DC: American Psychological Association.

Maryland Department of Housing and Community Development. (2016). EmPOWER Maryland low income energy efficiency program 2016. Accessed 14 June 2016.

Minnesota Housing Finance Agency. Rehabilitation loan/emergency and accessibility loan program (2016). Accessed 14 June 2016.

Poole, J. C., Dobson, K. S., & Pusch, D. (2017). Childhood adversity and adult depression: The protective role of psychological resilience. *Child Abuse & Neglect, 64*, 89–100. https://doi.org/10.1016/j.chiabu.2016.12.

Robinson, P. J., Gould, D., & Strosahl, K. D. (2010). *Real behavior change in primary care. Strategies and tools for improving outcomes and increasing job satisfaction*. Oakland, CA: New Harbinger.

Schotanus-Dijkstra, M., ten Have, M., Lamers, S. M. A., de Graaf, R., & Bohlmeijer, E. T. (2017). The longitudinal relationship between flourishing mental health and mood, anxiety and substance use disorders. *European Journal of Public Health, 27*(3), 563–568. https://doi.org/10.1093/eurpub/ckw202

Seligman, M. E. P. (2012). *Flourish: A visionary new understanding of happiness and well-being*. New York, NY: Simon & Schuster.

Soots, L. (2018) The positive psychology people. http://www.thepositivepsychologypeople.com/
flourishing/. Accessed 18 June 2019.

Strosahl, K. D., Robinson, P. J., & Gustavsson, T. (2012). *Brief interventions for radical change: Principles and practice of focused acceptance and commitment therapy.* Oakland, CA: New Harbinger.

U.S. Department of Agriculture. Rural development. Single family housing repair loans & grants 2016. Available from: Single family housing repair loans & grants. Accessed 14 June 2016.

United States Department of Health. (2019). Office of disease prevention and health promotion. Healthy people 2020. https://www.healthypeople.gov. Accessed 20 June 2019.

Van der Weele, T. J. (2017). On the promotion of human flourishing. *Proceedings of the National Academy of Sciences, U.S.A., 31,* 8148–8156.

Chapter 4
Behavior Change in Primary Care: Assessment

Abbreviations

AAQ-II	Acceptance and Action Questionnaire-II
ACT	Acceptance and Commitment Therapy
BHC	Behavioral Health Clinician
PC	Primary Care
Clinician	Any healthcare clinician working in PC
DSM-5	Diagnostic and Statistical Manual of Mental Disorders-5
DUKE	Duke Health Profile
EHR	Electronic Health Record
FACT	Focused Acceptance and Commitment Therapy
LP	Liaison Psychiatrist
PIG	Pillars Assessment Guide
PAT	Pillars Assessment Tool
PCC	Primary Care Clinician
Ph	Pharmacist
PT	Physical Therapist

A new approach to assessment of behavioral health concerns is needed in primary care (PC), one that is engaging for patients and feasible for clinicians. Historically, assessment of psychological problems in primary care (PC) focused on identifying symptoms and matching them to a list to obtain a diagnosis from the Diagnostic and Statistical Manual of Mental Disorders-5 (DSM-5, American Psychiatric Association, 2016). A diagnosis was assumed to be important because it could suggest a specific treatment, the delivery of which would cure or at least improve the condition.

While this sounds straight forward, this approach has encountered many problems in implementation and has fallen short in efforts to alleviate suffering related to behavioral health problems. First, clinicians rarely have time to complete rule-out diagnostic interviews in brief primary care visits, and this results in less reliable diagnoses. Second, patients may feel uncomfortable with some questions and experience

P. J. Robinson, *Basics of Behavior Change in Primary Care*, SpringerBriefs
in Psychology, https://doi.org/10.1007/978-3-030-32050-8_4

discouragement rather than encouragement from the assessment process. Third, there are concerns about the inter-rater reliability of diagnoses made with the use of the DSM, even after extensive training and with time allowed for an extensive interviewing. These concerns date back to 1960's and whether field trials on the most recent version of the DSM demonstrate reliability better than earlier versions is controversial (Frances, 2012). A final concern about this approach to assessment is that the group of evidence-based behavioral treatments for a wide variety of diagnoses are remarkably similar. This leads many to question the relative value of conducting lengthy psychiatric assessments as they often do not contribute significantly to treatment precision.

This chapter offers an alternative approach to assessment for Primary Care Clinicians (PCCs), Behavioral Health Clinicians (BHCs), Liaison Psychiatrists (LPs), Pharmacists (Phs), Physical Therapists (PTs), and other staff working in PC settings. This new approach begins with an introduction designed to prepare patients to participate actively in the assessment. Readers will learn about the Contextual Interview Questions (Table 4.1), an alternative to a symptom-focused diagnostic interview and the Four-Square tool (Table 4.2) for conceptualizing an engaging behavioral experiment. Readers will also learn to use the FACT Pillars Assessment

Table 4.1 Contextual interview questions[a]

Life context: Love, work, play and health	
Love	Where do you live? With whom? How long have you been there? Are things okay at your home? Do you have loving relationships with your family or friends?
Work	Do you work? Study? If yes, what is your work? Do you enjoy it? If not working, are you looking for work? If not working and not looking for a job, how do your support yourself?
Play	What do you do for fun? For relaxation? For connecting with people in your neighborhood or community?
Health	Do you use tobacco products, alcohol, illegal drugs, social media? Do you exercise on a regular basis for your health? Do you eat well? Sleep well?
Problem context: The three T's	
Time	When did this start? How often does it happen? What happens before / after the problem? Why do you think it is a problem now?
Trigger	Is there anything—a situation or a person—that seems to set it off?
Trajectory	What's this problem been like over time? Have there been times when it was less of a concern? More of a concern? And recently…getting worse, better?
Workability Question	What have you tried (to address the problem)? How has that worked in the short run? In the long run or in the sense of being consistent with what really matters to you?

[a]Adapted from Robinson, Gould, & Strosahl, 2010.

Table 4.2 Four-square tool[a]

	Avoidance / Controls suffering	Approach / Supports flourishing
Actions		
Thoughts		
Emotions		
Sensations		

[a]Adapted from Strosahl, Robinson, & Gustavsson, 2012.

Tool (PAT) (Table 4.3) to evaluate patient strengths and weaknesses and brainstorm targets for change on the pillars of open, aware, and engaged. The chapter ends with a checklist of recommended strategies for readers to use to select targets for pursuing new assessment methods—methods that support radical behavior change.

Table 4.3 FACT Pillars Assessment Tool (PAT)

Use this tool to assess patient functioning in each pillar and to plan interventions that might be helpful.

1. What are the patient's strengths and weaknesses?

2. Is there a pillar that is a priority target for skill development at this point in time?

Open	Aware	Engaged
• Accepts distressing thoughts and feelings • Creates a safe observational distance from distressing thoughts and feelings • Uses experiences to inform behavior, rather than habits and rules	• Intentionally focuses on present moment experience • Uses self-reflective awareness to promote sensitivity to context • Can change perspectives on stories told about self and others	• Speaks about values with emotion, recalls moments of values-in-action, and accepts vulnerability that comes with caring • Plans and implements behavior change experiments that promote vitality
Strengths	**Strengths**	**Strengths**
Deficits	**Deficits**	**Deficits**
Targets	**Targets**	**Targets**

Starting a Conversation about Behavior Change

An assessment should begin with the clinician offering a patient an introduction that describes the purpose and structure of assessment. This explanation needs to inform the patient about assessment methods and time required. The following is an example of an introduction that a clinician might use to start a conversation about assessment.

In hearing you describe your concerns today, I am thinking that X (problem) is beginning to affect your sense of well-being. I want to complete a brief survey with you so that we know what your quality of life scores are right now; this will take about 3 minutes. We'll check on this again when you return to the clinic, so that we can see if the scores come up. After that, I will ask a lot of questions about your life as it is right now and the problem—the what, when, where, etc. This will take about five to 10 minutes. Then, we will put our heads together and come up with a plan. I think we can figure out a way to make things better for you.

A patient may complete the standardized assessment after the clinician's introduction, or the clinician may think it best to assist the patient in completing the assessment by interview. In some instances, particularly at follow-up visits, patients often complete the quality of life survey prior to the visit. This brief introduction script helps the patient understand the assessment process and the value of completing the survey.

Standardized Assessments

When it comes to use of surveys to assist with assessment, patient preferences are important. Patients prefer short surveys with questions that give them a better understanding of their situation. For example, questions about social activities, such as how often they talk with friends, or their ability to engage in a physical activity, such as climbing a flight of stairs, help a patient focus their attention on their daily or weekly behaviors. Measures of health-related quality of life are less likely to trigger patient experience of stigma related to mental health than surveys asking about symptoms, such as not liking yourself. Since patients want a high quality of life, use of a survey that provides patients with understandable scores encourages interest in using outcomes to monitor physical, mental, and social health. When the survey is re-administered at follow-up visits, patients are interested in learning about quantifiable change in a health measure after implementing a behavioral experiment.

The Duke Health Profile (DUKE) is an example of a brief measure of health-related quality of life with high acceptability to patients (Duke Family Medicine and Community Health Department, n.d.) . It includes 17 items and requires less than 5 minutes to complete, score and discuss. The DUKE is normed on primary care patients, and it is available in over two dozen languages. Scoring includes the option of giving patients feedback on 4 functioning scores: Physical Health, Mental Health, Social Health, and General Health. The scores range from 0–100, and higher scores indicate better functioning. Patients like the idea of trying to make their scores go up, like on a spelling test. Duke scoring takes a patient's age and gender into account, so patients of any age may expect to push their scores toward 100. Permission to use the DUKE is available through Duke University Family Medicine Department. The Duke Family Medicine and Community Health Department has developed other measures for PC, including the Duke Health Profile-8 (Duke-8) and the Duke Population Health Profile (Duke-PH, for details on all Duke scales see https://fmch. duke.edu/research/duke-health-measures).

Another option for estimating patient functioning is the PROMIS® (Patient-Reported Outcomes Measurement Information System). HealthMeasures is the official source of information for PROMIS® measures and is responsible for distribution of PROMIS measures (http://www.healthmeasures.net/explore-measurement-systems/promis). PROMIS® includes a set of measures that evaluate health in adults and children. It is designed for the general population and brief versions are available. Like the Duke, PROMIS® measures generate scores on Physical, Mental and Social Health. Developed and evaluated with funding from the National Institutes of Health (NIH), PROMIS® surveys are available in the public domain.

Use of the DUKE or PROMIS® support a biopsychosocial approach to assessment. In offering feedback on survey results, clinicians have an opportunity to acknowledge a patient's strength (e.g., "looks like your social health is pretty good – higher than your physical and mental health scores; that's a good sign") or recognize a patient for seeking care when all scores are low (e.g., "looks like life has been pretty hard on you lately"). As feedback typically occurs in the first few minutes of the assessment, it can be a clinician's first chance to intentionally strengthen the connection between themselves and the patient.

Rating Scale Questions

Three rating scale assessments are built into this functional approach to assessment (See Table 4.4). Patient ratings on problem severity, confidence in the planned behavioral experiment, and helpfulness of the visit assist clinicians in making moment-to-moment decisions during the course of the interview. Patients use a scale of 1–10 to respond to the questions. The rating scale questions can be incorporated into Electronic Health Records (EHRs) to aid clinicians with quick assessments of change in follow-up visits.

The first rating scale question asked in the interview is the problem severity question: "On a scale of 1 to 10, where one is not a problem and 10 is a very big problem, how big of a problem is "x" for you at this time?"

This question is asked in the initial visit and at all follow-up visits. Problem severity estimates the patient's level of psychosocial distress concerning the problem. Big problems create high distress and enhance the patient's level of interest in seeking help. If there is little distress about the problem, the patient may be less motivated to change their behavior in relationship to the problem.

Table 4.4 Rating scale questions [a]

1. How big of a problem is *x*?   1 = not a problem and 10 = a very big problem
2. How confident are you that you will *do* this experiment?   1 = not confident and 10 = very confident
3. How helpful was this visit?   1 = not helpful and 10 = very helpful

In the follow-up interview, the problem severity rating question is one of the first questions asked by the clinician. The patient's response informs the assessment strategy for that visit. If the problem is improving, the clinician will ask for details about the improvement – what, how, who noticed, etc. When outcomes are less positive, the clinician will probe for specific indicators of the problem improving somewhat, remaining unchanged, or worsening. Additionally, the clinician will try to identify behaviors the patient used to keep the problem from worsening, etc. When a problem is not improving, the clinician may revisit the problem and pursue further functional assessment to inform a stronger conceptualization for a new behavioral experiment. Whether the problem is improving or not, the clinician also explores the patient's experience with the behavior change plan in follow-up visits, as well as the possibility that the patient may have conducted other experiments in an effort to address the problem.

The second rating scale question concerns patient confidence in following through with the behavioral experiment formulated in the visit: "To what extent are you confident that you will do the experiment, on a scale where one is not confident and 10 is very confident?"

The clinician is hoping for a confidence rating of seven or higher. If less than seven, the clinician will explore what change to the plan would move the patient to a confidence rating of seven or higher. Patients may interpret this question to be about their confidence in the plan *changing* the problem. However, this is not the question. If this appears to be the patient's understanding, the clinician needs to clarify that the rating concerns only the patient's confidence in *doing* the plan. The clinician can then emphasize the importance of the patient trying something new to see how it works. This is a great time for the clinician to highlight the value of "failure" in a behavioral experiment, as it helps to clarify what is and what is not helpful. Chapter 5 provides more on the power of failure in behavior change.

The third rating scale question is the helpfulness question: "To what extent has this visit been helpful? Use a scale of one = not helpful to 10 = very helpful to let me know."

The clinician asks this question at the end of the visit and may introduce it by reminding the patient, "As you may remember, I told you at the beginning of the visit that my job is be helpful and now I need to know how helpful this visit has been for you." While this may be a little socially awkward for the clinician and patient, it shows that the clinician respects the patient and encourages honesty and openness in their relationship. When giving the helpfulness rating, some patients will spontaneously tell the clinician what was helpful in the visit, and this information may sometimes contain surprises. Asking this question consistently helps clinicians become better clinicians. When a patient gives a rating of less than seven, it is a good idea for the clinician to ask the patient what they could have done that would have been more helpful. The helpfulness question, like the other rating scale questions, is asked in the initial and all follow-up visits.

Contextual Interview Questions

Use of questions suggested in Table 4.1 (Contextual Interview Questions), encourages development of a strong relationship with the patient during the course of assessment, because of their focus on the patient's experience and understanding. Patients like to be seen as experts on themselves and they tend to trust a plan that results from a clinician taking the time to understand the patient's point of view. The goals of contextual interviewing are to obtain information about the patient's life context and to complete a functional evaluation of the problem. Sometimes, the clinician does not need to assess the life context because they already know the patient well.

At other times, the clinician may have a busy schedule and lack the time needed to complete both sections (i.e., life and problem). When time is limited, even if the patient is new to the clinician, it may be best for the clinician to focus on problem context questions and complete the life context questions in a future visit. While this may result in a less precise behavioral experiment, it is best to help the patient develop a plan than to suggest that they return on a different day.

The Contextual Interview Questions (Table 4.1) help clinicians to be time-effective in completing functional assessments. The wording of questions can be changed to accommodate cultural and other factors, such as the patient's developmental context. For example, rather than asking questions about work, a clinician would ask an 8-year-old questions about school, such as, "What grade are you in? Do you like your teachers?"

Not all questions are necessary in all interviews; the list is suggestive. That being said, it is a well-thought-out list and one that clinicians are wise to use while learning the skills of functional assessment. The yes / no format helps clinicians quickly obtain information for a broad understanding of the patient's current life circumstances.

Participating in the contextual interview is a cognitively demanding task for patients and patient behavior in this demand situation provides information about the patient's psychological flexibility. To what extent is the patient able to maintain their attention on the questions? Does the patient engage in questions related to their values or answer in a superficial way? What are the patient's non-verbal behaviors communicating? Does the patient look away or fidget with their phone? Does a patient tell long stories?

Using a standard list of questions as a reference helps clinicians to ask the questions while simultaneously considering clues as the patient's overall psychological flexibility. During the course of the contextual interview, a clinician listens to the patient's answers and observes the patient's behavior to better understand the patient's level of psychological flexibility. As you will recall, Focused Acceptance and Commitment Therapy (FACT) and the pillars of psychological flexibility (i.e., open, aware, engaged) were introduced in Chap. 3 (for more information, see Robinson, Gould & Strosahl, 2010; Strosahl, Robinson & Gustavsson, 2012). This chapter provides a tool for gauging a patient's psychological flexibility and identifying ways to promote more flexible responding (see Table 4.3 FACT Pillars Assessment Tool, PAT).

To begin the life context questions, a clinician might say, "To understand your situation, I need information about different areas of your life, so I'll be asking a lot of questions for the next 5 minutes." The pace of the interview for life context questions is fast. The clinician explores home, work, play and health issues, looking at how they relate to the patient's problem. Many questions are best asked in a close-ended format. Sometimes, patient answers suggest a need for follow-up questions, but it is important for the clinician to avoid getting side-tracked and to continue to pursue the goal of getting a "snap shot" of the four areas: love, work, play and health. This section of the Contextual Interview has a social flavor, and most patients feel more comfortable in talking about their lives and daily routines before moving to the problem. Many patients relax and shift towards a perspective on their problem that is more curious and less distressed.

Contextual questions encourage patients to look at the problem from a functional point of view, and this is a new frame for investigating the problem for most patients. Questions about time, triggers, and trajectory provide clues about contextual factors that maintain the behavior. The very process of answering the questions provides patients with a chance to modify their outlook or to add to the story about the problem, such that they may be more able to experience compassion for themselves or others related to the problem. As the problem context interview moves toward exploration of the patient's attempts to solve the problem, the pace of the interview slows and the clinician may find moments of silence to be important in encouraging the patient to think more deeply and to focus on emotions and the way they are experienced in the body.

Workability and Values Clarification

The questions associated with workability set the stage for behavior change: "What have you tried (to address the problem)? How has that worked in the short run? In the long run or in the sense of being consistent with what really matters to you?"

Often, patients are continuing to try the same solutions to their problems, even though their solutions provide only short-term relief for the problem and may have unintended costs. A person who works in a stressful job and uses alcohol to relax after work provides a good example. The single beer of a few years ago has become a 6-pack, and their relationship with their partner is stressed to the point of breaking. Engaging patients in a meaningful conversation about their values may provide important motivation for their transforming avoidance behaviors into approach behaviors.

Clinicians can use of these four guidelines to intensify their conversations with patients about values, and the role that values are playing in the problem. Often, the problem that the patient brings to the clinician is a problem because the patient cares a great deal about something related to it.

1. Ask the patient *what matters* and *who matters* in regard to the problem. These simple questions tend to elicit more heartfelt answers than simply asking a patient what values are related to the problem.
2. Ask the patient to describe a situation when they felt very connected with the value they perceive to be of importance in solving their current problem. For example, a patient might say that it is important to show respect in how they address a difficult relationship with a work colleague. When asked for an example of "respecting in action" the patient might offer something like the following.

> Well, that would be when my father had a stroke. I had been frustrated with him for a long time and felt he didn't really understand me. He had been critical of me and I had been angry with him for years. Yet, we never gave up, and I don't believe either of us ever really wanted to hurt the other. When he was in the hospital, I went to him and told him that I appreciated the fact that he cared about me and that I knew that being my father had been difficult for him at times. I told him that I respected him for trying to help me be a better person. You know, we both shed a few tears and I felt a stronger connection with him then than I had in years.

In moving to a specific example of valuing-in-action, patients can tap into the emotional power of values and use it as fuel for behavior change.

3. Ask the patient to bring the memory of valuing-in-action to their present moment experience. Here, the clinician might ask the patient, "Are you experiencing some of the feelings you had then now at this very moment, as you consider respect? Can you show me how your face might have looked when you were there with your Dad? And as you take on that expression, what starts to happen in your body? Where do you feel respect in your body?" These questions may help strengthen the person's connection with what matters and who matters.
4. Encourage the patient to stay with the feeling of vulnerability that comes with a strong connection to a value. A patient's eyes may moisten, or they may cry when connecting with a strongly held value. Clinicians need not talk a lot about this connection and instead slow down perhaps encouraging a patient by saying, "I hope you will allow yourself a moment to experience what you are feeling. This is important". The extent to which a person can experience their own vulnerability is important because vulnerability is a necessary part of caring and pursuing a vital life centered around what matters and who matters.

The Four-Square Tool

As you may recall from Chap. 3, many patients challenged by making changes to their behavior are caught in a struggle between avoiding what they don't want and approaching what matters. This chapter introduces the Four-Square Tool (Table 4.2) which invites clinicians to conceptualize behaviors discovered in a functional assessment as serving either an approach/value-consistent function or an avoidance/control function. In our functional assessment, thoughts, feelings, and sensations are considered to be internal behaviors or those occurring inside the person. Actions that a person takes and that could potentially be observed are external behaviors. The Four-Square Tool is similar to the Approach-Avoidance Tool (Table 3.3) introduced in Chap. 3 but includes the concept of workability. The Four-Square Tool may be used for conceptualization purposes or as a clinical tool in working with patients. Later in this chapter, the Four-Square Tool is demonstrated in a clinician's work with three patients.

Contextual Assessment Checklist.

The contextual interview concludes when the clinician knows the answers to questions listed in The Contextual Assessment Checklist (Table 4.5). These questions identify critical information for clinicians to use in transitioning to behavior change planning with the patient. If unsure, clinicians are wise to ask a few more questions to clarify the answers to these four important questions.

1. What is the patient doing to address the problem?
2. How are their solutions are working?
3. What matters and who matters to the patient?
4. What might the patient do in a world where anything was possible?

Table 4.5 Contextual assessment checklist

Do I know:
1. What the patient is doing to address the problem
2. How their solutions are working
3. What matters and who matters to the patient
4. What the patient might do in a world where anything was possible

Values always play a role in the problem; however, a patient's connection with the values may not be strong. Likewise, patients are problem-solvers, and they are always trying to address their problems. The extent to which they are not succeeding is directly related to their level of psychosocial distress; the greater the struggle, the greater the distress level. Many times, patients are trying to address the problem by avoiding or controlling it – not thinking about it, trying not to feel it, or doing things that help them not think about it or feel it. Perhaps the problem involves attachment to a "rule" that gets in the way of what a person wants. For example, "Don't show your weakness; if you do, people will walk all over you" is a rule that would wreak havoc for a person who is trying to solve the problem of loneliness by developing an intimate relationship.

Answers to item four on the Contextual Assessment Checklist (i.e., What would the patient do in a world where anything was possible?) help the clinician estimate the patient's ability to take a perspective of possibility on the problem. If a patient is able to make this shift, they may readily see options for behavior change. If it is more difficult for the patient, they may benefit from discussion of avoided thoughts and feelings and the role they play in the person's life. Thoughts can function as bullies in a person's life (e.g., "You are damaged goods; no one will want to be with you if they really know you".) and feelings may be bullies, too (e.g., fear associated with the memory of an accident where a person sustained an injury that led to development of chronic pain). Clinicians may also work more on clarifying values and strengthening the patient's connections with values in an effort to support development of a perspective of possibility and willingness to engage in a new behavior. When done well, the contextual interview sets the stage for behavior change. In Chap. 5, readers learn more about how to help patients whose lives are made more complex by psychological inflexibility.

Case Examples

The contextual interview provides a platform for understanding the many varieties of psychological pain and suffering that primary care patients experience. Bob, Amy, and Mary are three primary care patients seeking help from a clinician working in a primary care setting. A contextual assessment will help us understand their difficulties and conceptualize ways to help. While their life contexts differ, they have a lot in common—they want to live meaningful lives; they have difficult things happening in their lives, and they are hurting. Their efforts to solve their problems involve avoidance and interfere with their efforts to live the lives they want and deserve.

In Chap. 3, readers learned about Acceptance and Commitment Therapy (ACT) and Focused Acceptance and Commitment Therapy (FACT) (Robinson, Gould & Strosahl, 2010; Strosahl, Robinson & Gustavsson, 2012). FACT offers assessment and intervention strategies that are helpful to patients with psychological and medical problems. ACT proposes a distinction between pain and suffering (Hayes, Strosahl, & Wilson, 2012). Specifically, ACT suggests that pain is a part of life; there is loss, illness, violence, a lack of justice, etc. *Psychological pain* is a very human response to these challenges of living. However, *psychological suffering* is added-on to the experience of psychological pain, it is the pain that comes with avoidance of psychological pain.

Focused ACT describes suffering as the the struggle to avoid directly experiencing and accepting pain that comes into one's life (Robinson, Gould, & Strosahl, 2010; Strosahl, Robinson, & Gustavsson, 2012). From birth, humans experience various unwanted and difficult experiences, with some originating from the external environment and some deriving from a person's unique human make-up. External experiences that trigger distress may include physical events (e.g., a significant rise or decrease in temperature, scarcity of food) and social experiences (e.g., verbal or physical aggression from another person or group of persons, exclusion from valued group activities). One's genetic makeup and life experience to date come together to create one's current resources, including thoughts, feelings, sensations, and behavioral proclivities and these come together to either mitigate or aggravate the response to painful life experiences and suffering.

Learning the skills associated with psychological flexibility may help Amy, Bob, and Mary live more meaningful lives, but not pain-free lives. The FACT perspective on Amy, Bob, and Mary is that they are "stuck but not broken". Clinicians do not need to make their difficult thoughts and feelings go away, but instead help them relate to them differently.

Figure 4.1 (FACT Pillars of Psychological Flexibility) describes the key qualities of psychological flexibility for each of the three pillars. Print this guide and use it as a reference as you read through the remainder of this chapter and perhaps during a

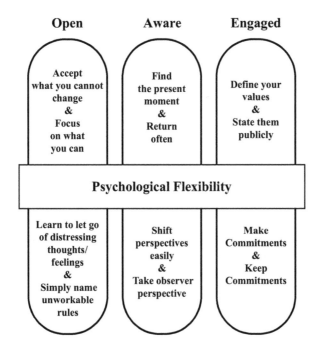

Fig. 4.1 FACT pillars of flexibility

day in the clinic. Referencing these descriptors helps clinicians adopt a conceptual frame for observing patients during contextual interviews. Let's look at Amy, Bob, and Mary and the problems they are facing in their lives and how psychological flexibility influences their response to their problems. In Chap. 5, Amy, Bob, and Mary return in illustrations of behavior change interventions.

Amy: Trauma and Health Risk Behavior

Amy is a 15-year-old sophomore in high school. She lives in low income housing with her mother and younger brother, Sam. Amy's mother works nights in a factory, and Amy takes care of Sam at night, getting him to bed and getting him up and off to school in the mornings. On weekends, she works part-time in a pharmacy, stocking supplies. She is saving some of her money and has hopes of going to college to study writing. Amy's father died of a heart attack about a year and a half ago. Her parents divorced when she was 12. Amy was a "daddy's girl" and she missed him a lot after he left her home and she worried about his health and his "getting into trouble because he was drinking too much". Amy's father was an alcoholic and his health declined sharply after the divorce.

Six months ago, Amy was sexually assaulted by an older boy living in her neighborhood. He came upon her when she was sitting in an unfinished home near her apartment building. He told her that if she ever told anyone, something bad would happen to her brother. Amy never told anyone, and she tries not to think about it. When she feels anxious or upset, she tries to focus on her school work, her job and taking care of Sam. If her feelings becoming overwhelming, she takes a razor blade and makes a few cuts on her forearm. This seems to help her snap back to reality, and she is able to do what she needs to do.

Amy started smoking her father's cigarettes occasionally when she was 11, and now she has an older friend who buys her a pack or two a week. When she is able to spend a weekend night with an older girlfriend from work, they meet up with other older teenagers and drink beer. Amy has been drunk a few times, and she thought it felt pretty good— "like nothing to worry about". She's skipped school a few times to hang out with some of her friends who are not in school anymore, but has never been caught.

Bob: Life Stress and Difficulties with Self-Management of Chronic Disease

Bob is married, a father to one son, and employed in a local auto supply store. He has held his job for over 20 years and knows the store "like the back of my hand". A couple of months ago, the store owner and Bob's long-term friend, Les, let him know that he planned to sell the store to an auto supply chain because of his health problems. He told Bob that he wasn't able to guarantee that his job would remain the same when the new owners took over. Bob thought it would be too much trouble to find a new job, so he stayed and hoped for the best.

A new manager started in the store a couple of weeks ago, and Bob understood that he would be the person to decide whether Bob would be let go or retained and possibly moved to a different position. Bob had tried to be cordial and helpful to the new manager, but he had a manner about him that rubbed Bob the wrong way. Shortly after the new manager started, Les stopped working at the store. This was a loss for Bob, as Les was a good friend.

For some reason, knowing about Les having health problems made Bob worry more about his own health. Bob was overweight and his blood pressure and cholesterol had been problems for a while. His wife, Loretta, a bookkeeper, had tried to get him to eat better and start exercising for years. As stress increased at work, Bob dropped all efforts to improve his lifestyle habits. Recently, Loretta ended an argument with a statement that hurt, "Go get some of those pills your sister takes. Maybe they'll help you stop being such a grump all the time". He avoided Loretta more after work and spent more time watching sports and eating take-out food. He told Loretta, "I will eat whatever I want to whenever I want and as much as I want!"

Mary: Grief and Demoralization

Mary likes her job as a clerk in an elementary school office. She's worked there 11 years and enjoys answering the phones, doing paper work, and, most of all, helping the children. Her husband died 9 years ago. She struggled for a while after his death but then slowly built a new life. She became a regular at church and enjoyed volunteer work in the church library. She joined a quilting circle that made little quilts for premature babies born at the local hospital.

Family was important to Mary. Her two adult children lived in different states, and she reached out to them weekly with a phone call. She also wrote them letters and sent them small gifts on a regular basis. Her daughter had never married, and her son had married and then divorced. The son had a daughter, but he did not have custody of the girl. Mary called and wrote the grand-daughter, Lucy, and Lucy's mother. Their relationship was amicable, and Lucy had come for week-long stays with Mary for the past two summers.

Mary's enthusiasm for life was once again shattered a year ago when she learned that her son, William, had died. Always sensitive and frequently sick as a child, William had struggled with back pain for many years, and it had seemed to worsen after his divorce 3 years ago. She knew his doctor had tried to change his medications for pain and that this had been difficult for him, but she had no idea that William had ever used street drugs. She was horrified to hear that it was a street drug for pain that cost him his life. Her daughter came for a short period of time and helped her organize the funeral. They moved William's belongings out of his apartment and into a bedroom at Mary's. After the funeral, Mary stopped going to church except very occasionally. She felt too tired to go to the quilting group and preferred to stay home and watch old movies. She continued to work but felt exhausted at work and looked forward to the end of the day.

Mary questioned why she was left to live out her old age with such pain and loneliness. Because family was so important to her, she did call Lucy, now eight, every Sunday. However, the little girl was not always available for these calls and that hurt. When Mary's daughter called her, Mary was cordial but avoided talking about William, dismissing her with comments like, "What's done is done; there's nothing to be said". She left Williams's belongings packed in boxes in the bedroom where they'd been moved after the funeral; she didn't open the door to that room. Over time, Mary ate less and slept less and the principal of the school where she worked expressed concern about her health and suggested that she see her doctor.

Amy, Bob, and Mary have encountered painful experiences in life –violence, job stress, relationship problems, health problems, and loss. They've struggled with recognizing and accepting their very difficult feelings of fear, rage, anger, loss, and sadness, and they are trying to cope with the pain by getting away from it—they are experiencing psychological suffering. Their "get-away" efforts rob them of energy needed to pursue what they care about. Amy wants to be independent and successful—a writer. Bob wants to be helpful to people and to be close with his wife. Mary wants to help the school children, connect with her daughter and granddaughter, and re-kindle her spiritual beliefs. Rather than changing their behavior to pursue what matters, they appear to be at risk of continuing with short-term solutions that tap down their suffering.

Pillars of Psychological Flexibility

Greater psychological flexibility enhances the ability to accept and understand pain and difficulties that arise in the normal course of living a human life, such as those Amy, Bob and Mary are experiencing. With greater flexibility, they will come to spend less time resisting or suppressing their problems and more time and energy doing what matters most! They will attend to their experience in the present moment, make choices that support their health, and learn from the results of small experiments involving new behaviors.

How clinicians assess psychological flexibly depends on the purpose of their assessment. Readers learned about the Acceptance and Action Questionnaire-II in Chap. 3 (Bond, Hayes, Baer, Carpenter, Guenole, et al., 2011, see Table 3.2), and it may be a useful survey for some patients and provide a general idea about the extent to which a patient is focused on trying to control or avoid problems. An assessment approach that helps clinicians identify targets for changing psychological flexibility is a valuable component of the assessment-intervention package.

The Pillars Assessment Tool The FACT Pillars Assessment Tool (PAT, Table 4.3) is such a tool and it invites clinicians to identify patient strengths and weaknesses in each of the three pillars of psychological flexibility—open, aware, and engaged. The PAT also encourages clinicians to set targets for enhancing psychological flexibility. The PAT may also be helpful for tracking patient change in levels of flexibility over time and could be shared with some patients as a component of treatment planning. It may be particularly useful for clinicians working with patients with more complexities who have experienced multiple traumas. Multiple traumas may hamper the ability to be open, aware, and engaged. However, patients who have survived many adverse events in their childhood have strengths—they are survivors! The PAT encourages clinicians to identify these strengths and to use them to support greater psychological flexibility over time, even in difficult contexts that trigger old habits. In Chap. 5, readers will learn to use the FACT Pillars Intervention Guide (PIG, Table 5.1) to promote psychological flexibility in moment-to-moment interactions with patients.

Putting It All Together

This section provides readers with an opportunity to see the tools introduced in this chapter in the context of care delivery. Interactions between clinicians and patients help readers perceive the subtleties of conducting engaging life context interviews and productive problem context interviews. Additionally, this section provides examples of using assessment information to conceptualize (1) targets for improving psychological flexibility (using the FACT Pillars Assessment Tool, PAT, Table 4.9) and (2) targets for the design of powerful behavioral experiments (using the Four-Square Tool, Table 4.13).

Amy

Reviewing segments of the clinician's interview with Amy provides an opportunity to highlight qualities of an engaging, effective life context interview. Most often, this will be the in the first part of a functional assessment, as it is social in nature and most patients expect to visit with healthcare clinicians about the general circumstances of their lives. Amy's mother brought her to the clinic after she received a call from the school saying that Amy had left school at lunch and that they wondered if the mother knew where she was. When confronted by her mother, Amy said she left school because she wasn't feeling well and that she had gone to a friend's house to rest. The mother was upset because she had asked Amy not to hang out with that particular person, as she had dropped at of school and seemed "troubled". Amy agreed to see the clinician, as she really did feel a little under the weather at this point.

Clinician: Hi, Amy. I haven't seen you in a long time. Are you still living with your mother and brother?

Amy: Yes.

Clinician: Is everything okay at home?

Amy: Yep. Mom works nights, and I take care of Sam. That goes well, but sometimes I don't get enough sleep. Maybe that's what's wrong with me.

Clinician: Okay. So sometimes you are tired. Do you make it to school most days?

Amy: Yes, nearly always. My grades are good, and I'm saving money so that maybe
I can go to college. I have a part-time job on weekends.

Clinician: Well, good for you. What do you do?

Amy: I stock shelves at the pharmacy on A Street, all of the bath, body, household
products-all that and then I do some cleaning. 16 hours and pay is okay.

Clinician: That's super; you've always impressed me as a smart and capable young
woman, and I think you'll do well in college. How are you doing in the "friends"
department? Anyone special in your life?

Amy: No, I don't have a boyfriend if that's what you mean. I don't have time for
that, and I don't really trust that many guys. I have some girlfriends and some older
guys that I just hang out with when I can.

Clinician: What do you all like to do?

Amy: Well you know, you won't tell my Mom, will you? We party, listen to music,
watch movies. They drink alcohol and smoke cigarettes.

Clinician: Do you think your Mom would approve?

Amy: No, and I don't want to upset her. She's already stressed out … worries way
too much.

Clinician: Don't want to be a bother?

Amy: Correct.

Clinician: Are you experimenting with drugs and alcohol?

Amy: No, drugs scare me. I've tried alcohol and tobacco – don't want to get hooked
on it though.

Clinician: Good for you. You have a good brain, Amy, and you are taking care of it.
What do you want to study at college?

Amy: I don't know … I think writing, but maybe sociology, too. I'm taking that at
school now and I like it. I like history, and I like writing poems. I used to go to a
place over by the old water tower where they were building some homes and well
it was a special place to write. But now, I just write at home at night mostly when
it's quiet. Maybe I'll be a teacher; I like some of the teachers at my school.
They're nice to me, smart, and you get the sense that they care about what they're
doing.

Clinician: Well, I think you would be an awesome teacher, Amy, but I hope you'll
consider writing and sociology, too and … even medicine. You know, we need
more doctors and nurses here and there's a lot of teaching in good medical care
and opportunities to write, too. Just a few more questions about your lifestyle?
Do you eat okay?

Amy: Pretty good. School lunches. I try to make something fresh for Sam and me
for dinner, and I make a plate for Mom to have when she gets home. She's really
big on vegetables.

In a few minutes, the clinician has gained an understanding of Amy's current life circumstances. The clinician adjusted the Contextual Interview questions so that they worked for an adolescent. Also, the clinician recognized and affirmed Amy's attempts to care for her health and to pursue her dreams. The clinician was already anticipating ways to incorporate Amy's strengths into a behavior change plan that might be helpful to her. She wanted to be independent, she could see herself in a career that she liked, she loved her brother and mother, and she seemed smart and capable of persevering. The clinician understood that Amy was lacking important social resources, namely more quality time with her mother and nurturing adults. The clinician knew that Amy's parents were divorced and that her father had died. As the clinician had been Amy's father's primary care clinician (PCC), the PCC also knew about the father's alcoholism and the extent to which this had troubled him and his family prior to his death. The clinician understood that Amy had already experienced several traumatic events in her young life and had a concern about her sense of safety, given her brief comment about not trusting men.

The clinician shifted easily from life context to the problem context, and Amy was ready for this discussion, as she was feeling understood and safe.

Clinician: So, what is the problem that brings you in today?

Amy: Well, I left school without getting Mom's permission or checking in at the office, so I'm in a bit of trouble with Mom and the school.

Clinician: How big of a problem is this for you, Amy? Like on a scale of one, it is not a problem, and 10, it is a very big problem.

Amy: Probably a 7 or 8 because I don't want it to bring my grades down and I don't want Mom to stress out.

Clinician: Now, when you're thinking about this problem, how do you feel?

Amy: A little sad and a little scared. It was stupid to leave like that.

Clinician: Did anything happen just before you decided to leave school?

Amy: Actually, something did happen. I was listening to two girls talking in the shower room and one was saying she was going to go out with this older man, Pete, on the weekend. I felt really sick inside because I know him and he is a mean dude. I just felt really weak and like I might throw up, so I dressed and walked out of the school. Then I ran all the way to Laura's house. Mom doesn't like her but she's really nice to me.

Clinician: Have you had that kind of "sick inside" feeling before?

Amy: Yes, and I hate it. When it happens, I just try to do something else – anything to get rid of it.

Clinician: Amy, if that feeling had a voice, what do you think it would say?

Amy: I don't know, probably "help"?

Clinician: Good, that's what I'm here for and I'm listening.. . . and just one more question, Amy, do you feel that you are safe from the mean dude, Pete?

Amy indicated that she did feel safe and that she was glad to have someone like the PCC to talk to. In less than 10 minutes, the clinician had used the Contextual Interview Questions to help Amy find a way to acknowledge her feelings and ask for help from an adult who could help. A tricky part of the contextual interview is

Table 4.6 Amy's four-square (Example)

	Not Workable	Workable
Actions	Walking away from school without talking to an adult Using alcohol with older friends Using alcohol to the point of intoxication Smoking Awake at night	Seeking care from clinician Working part time Saving money for college Completing homework and studying Attending school most of the time Caring for her brother Cooking for the family Writing poetry Using words to describe feelings
Thoughts Feelings Sensations	I'm not safe. I have to be careful. I can't tell other people about what happened to me. It's not safe to ask for help. Maybe it's all my fault. Don't' bother people. Fear. Sadness Loses focus of attention when triggered Fatigue	Loves her family Values self-expression and creativity Believes she can help others / teach Connects with her feelings Able to stay with a difficult feeling Values quiet time

defining of the problem of concern. At the beginning of the problem context inter-view, the problem definition was being in trouble with the school and her mother. A few minutes later, the definition changed to "feeling sick inside". Given the previous information Amy had shared about not trusting guys and not wanting a boyfriend, the clinician was seeing Amy's behavior in the context of trauma—when she felt unsafe and overwhelmed, she ran. This would work in the context of being among people that were currently threatening your safety, but it would not work well in the context of attending a physical education class. Running was also not going to help Amy complete high school or go to college.

Let's take a look at how the contextual interview information can be evaluated and used to conceptualize an intervention for Amy. The Four-Square analysis yields a long list of workable actions and workable thoughts, feelings, and sensations (See Table 4.6, Amy's Four Square). Amy has many strengths and they buffer the impact of the difficult things that have happened in her life. However, she is at a critical moment in her life, where she could easily become stuck in actions that help her avoid very painful thoughts, feelings, sensations, and memories, particularly those related to the possible recent assault.

Before moving to Bob, let's also take a look at what Amy's PAT might look like (See Table 4.7, Amy's PAT). As can be seen, Amy has strengths in all areas and the pillar that is perhaps most important to address in working with Amy's current prob-lem is that of openness. The PAT target priority would be experiments that help Amy detect triggers for leaving school, find a tender way to respond to the "sick feeling", and cultivate new skills for creating an immediate sense of safety. Certainly, other targets are possible, including design of experiments that give her an opportu-nity to talk more about her values and goals with adults who can support them.

Table 4.7 Amy's PAT (Example)

Open	Aware	Engaged
• Accepts distressing thoughts and feelings • Creates a safe observational distance from distressing thoughts and feelings • Uses experiences to inform behavior, rather than habits and rules	• Intentionally focuses on present moment experience • Uses self-reflective awareness to promote sensitivity to context • Can change perspectives on stories told about self and others	• Speaks about values with emotion, recalls moments of values-in-action, and accepts vulnerability that comes with caring • Plans and implements behavior change experiments that promote vitality
Strengths	**Strengths**	**Strengths**
Some strength evidenced by willingness to talk somewhat openly with clinician Possible strength of using poetry-writing to create a safe observational distance from painful thoughts and feelings	Some strength evidenced by ability to see herself in a future context	Definite area of strength: Speaks clearly about values, demonstrates ability to show love by caring for Sam and her mother
Deficits	**Deficits**	**Deficits**
Clearly unable to tolerate painful memories (possibly sexual assault and perhaps other traumas) when triggered	Unsure. Could explore ability to focus attention on the present moment in future contacts	
Targets	**Target**	**Targets**
Assist with ability to detect triggers, relate to pain with compassion, new skills for creating an immediate sense of safety		Increase frequency of writing about what matters Increase rates of talking with others (e.g., teachers, mother) about what matters

Bob

Bob finally made an appointment with a clinician in PC because it was getting harder and harder for him to get to work in the morning. Bob didn't see the point in talking about his problems and he didn't believe in pills that made you happy. Bob dreaded having his blood pressure taken and he hated to get on the scales. He couldn't remember when he was supposed to have seen the doctor about his labs, but he thought it was a while back and seemed to recall ignoring several reminder calls, so he anticipated a bit of a lecture. His former clinician had retired several years ago and his new one was young. He questioned whether or not they had enough experience with medicine to know how to manage his health problems and wondered if they were "just guessing" about his medicines. The clinician began the interview with a summary of what they knew about Bob's life from their previous visits.

Clinician: Hi, Bob. It's good to see you. I just want to check in on your home and work situations to make sure I have the latest information. You are still living with your wife and you are still at the auto store, right?

Bob: Yes, that's right today, but I don't know about tomorrow.

Clinician: How's that, Bob?

Bob: The store's been sold and I'm not sure if the new people will want me. Frankly, I don't think they know what they're doing, and they might not know what an asset I am to the store.

Clinician: I would find that pretty unsettling. I mean I like my job and I care about what other people think about the quality of my work. Is your wife helpful with this situation? How about your son?

Bob: My wife thinks I need some of those happy pills you guys give out to everybody.

Clinician: (smiling) How about your son? Anybody on Team Bob?

Bob: I don't want to bother him with my problems; sophomore year of college is hard enough. He's still studying business; he's smart.

Clinician: Sounds like you're trying to handle this by yourself, Bob. Are you making any headway?

Bob: Well, I've looked around a little for other jobs – like a similar job but at another store, and, from what I've seen, I think I'd have to take a big pay cut. I can't be between jobs now because we need my income to keep our son in school. It'd be hard to get by on less money, but I guess we could. To tell you the truth, it's hard to think about leaving. You know I've been there for 20 years; got that job when my son was 9 months old.

Clinician: You sound sad, Bob, and I understand that. You are the kind of person that cares about customers and co-workers and commitment. This change is being forced on you, and it hurts to think of letting go.

Bob: Well, you got that right. Guess they teach you to talk good like that in doctoring school, huh?

Clinician: I want to say things well, Bob, and I'm genuinely worried about you. You said you've looked around a bit; are there other things you are trying or thinking of trying?

Bob: I'm trying to be nice to the new manager, so that he'll pick me. And I'm watching a lot of baseball, and, if the Mariners were doing better, I think I'd probably be drinking less beer. I haven't applied for any other jobs if that's what you mean; I don't want to go to all that trouble if I don't have to.

Clinician: Do you feel like you're building a working relationship with the new manager?

Bob: A little. He's kind of know-it-all type guy, but he doesn't know much about this store and our inventory. He has to ask me questions. Of course, I nearly always have the answers. I know that store like the back of my hand.

Clinician: Hmm, that's interesting, Bob. You're doing something that's pretty difficult. Like you can feel sad about all the changes and at the same time still be helpful to the new manager, right?

Bob: I never thought about it that way, but I guess, yes, I do, at least sometimes. Mostly though, I feel upset at work and then I just look at the clock and count the hours I have to put in before I can go home. Guess I need to try to figure out how to be helpful when I'm in a bad mood, huh?

Clinician: That's a difficult thing to do, but I think it's a good direction to pursue.

Bob: I thought you'd be on me about my weight and my blood pressure and cholesterol. You're being pretty nice today.

Clinician: Those things are important, too, Bob, but I think addressing your work
   situation is the priority today. Do you agree?

Bob: Yes, for sure. But I do want you to know that I'm taking all those pills you gave
   me; I take them every day.

Clinician: That's awesome, Bob, stay with your medicines. You care about your
   health, and we can look at other small things you can do to protect it over time.
   Today, I am hoping that we can firm up a plan for the stressful job situation, your
   understandable sadness, and the worries you have about money and your job in
   the future.

In this contextual interview, the clinician made a quick shift from the life context
to the problem context by following the patient's lead. They sensed Bob's discomfort
with seeking care and knew that he had not come for requested follow-ups in the past
6 months, even with multiple phone and email reminders from the clinic. The clinician wanted to engage him in care and that meant addressing what mattered most to
him. If the clinician can help him develop a more approach-oriented direction to
work stress, that will possibly energize approach-oriented behavior related to his
physical health. Rather than lecture, the clinician affirmed Bob for caring about his
health and acknowledged the success evidenced by his medication adherence.

Let's take a look at how the contextual interview information can be evaluated
and used to conceptualize an intervention for Bob. The Four-Square analysis yields
a somewhat short list of workable actions and the clinician would like to see Bob
engaging in more value-consistent actions (See Table 4.8, Bob's Four-Square).
Thoughts and feelings about the importance of family and health are good assets for
fueling better engagement. However, Bob has a long list of unworkable thoughts,
feelings, and sensations and some easy to execute avoidance behaviors (i.e., beer

Table 4.8 Bob's four-square (Example)

	Not Workable	Workable
Actions	Drinking beer to get away from negative thoughts and feelings	Making an appointment to see the clinician
	Watching television to get away from his wife and negative thoughts and feelings	Going to work
		Being helpful to new manager
	Arguing with wife about lifestyle behaviors and health	Exploring new job possibilities
	Acting like everything is fine with his son	Taking his medications
Thoughts	This isn't fair.	Loves his wife and son
	I have to make the same amount of money.	I am a good provider.
	No one really understands my situation.	I can make small changes to protect my health.
	Getting a new job is too much trouble.	
	I don't want to think about this or my health.	My health is important to me.
	I can eat whatever I want to whenever I want to.	I am smart and capable.
		Caring about wife and son
Feelings	Sad, angry	
Sensations	?	

Table 4.9 Bob's PAT (Example)

Open	Aware	Engaged
• Accepts distressing thoughts and feelings • Creates a safe observational distance from distressing thoughts and feelings • Uses experiences to inform behavior, rather than habits and rules	• Intentionally focuses on present moment experience • Uses self-reflective awareness to promote sensitivity to context • Can change perspectives on stories told about self and others	• Speaks about values with emotion, recalls moments of values-in-action, and accepts vulnerability that comes with caring • Plans and implements behavior change experiments that promote vitality
Strengths	**Strengths**	**Strengths**
Some strength evidenced by ability to notice that he can feel sad and still be helpful to his new manager	Some strength evidenced by ability to be in the moment in the interview, to use humor in interacting with clinician	Definite area of strength: Speaks about values, demonstrates ability to show love by continuing to work and support son's studies
Deficits	**Deficits**	**Deficits**
Lacks skills for noticing difficult thoughts and feelings related to lifestyle behaviors and health Problematic avoidance behaviors related to arguing with wife, use of alcohol	Needs assistance with developing new perspectives on self-story	Difficulties with initiating and sustaining behavior changes to promote satisfying employment and to promote better health Would benefit from placing these changes in a values context, learning self-monitoring, being more able to encourage himself
Targets	**Target**	**Targets**
Assist with skills for detecting and accepting negative feelings at work, while engaging in helpful behaviors Find a way to honor his sadness and sense of loss	Encourage perspective of "possibility" (in a world where anything was possible ...) Encourage future perspective (if you were you and 5 years in the future and looking back at this point in time, what would you. ..) Help Bob tune into sensation in his body, be intentionally present	Increase job search activities Ask son to help with development of a resume Ask for meeting with new manager for the purpose of identifying more ways he could be helpful

and television). It's easy to see how he is stuck and finding it difficult to move forward in addressing his work situation proactively.

Before moving to Mary, let's also take a look at what Bob's PAT might look like (See Table 4.9, Bob's PAT). As can be seen, Bob has strengths and deficits in all areas and a variety of targets for improving his psychological flexibility are important. Given his tenuous engagement in healthcare, the clinician wants to give him options for exploring small changes, allowing him a choice. To do this, the clinician might say,

> Bob, there's a couple of ways to go here and I'm not sure what's right. On the one hand, you
> could go out and do something to directly address the job problem– things like schedule a

meeting with your boss to discuss ways you can be more helpful in the transition or even asking your son if he might help with a resume if you want to look at other jobs. On the other hand, I think it might be helpful for you to pause and get a handle on what's important about how you handle this transition. A helpful perspective might be imagining that you were looking back at today from 5 years in the future. What would you like to be seeing youself do to address this problem … what qualities would be important in how you handle the problem … different for different people … and helpful to know. Which of these directions makes sense to you? The action angle or the perspective angle?

By providing Bob with a choice, the clinician shows confidence in Bob and respect for his independence. The clinician's priority is to engage Bob in care at this point. When he is more engaged, other targets for enhancing his skills for working flexibly with problems of living and health challenges are possible.

Mary

Mary's clinician knew her well, and she was always glad to see Mary was on her schedule. The clinician was aware of Mary's challenging life circumstances, and she saw her as a "survivor". Before the visit, the clinician noted Mary's vitals and noticed that she had an unintended weight loss of over 10 pounds in the past 6 months. The weight loss was a concern, as Mary was now underweight. The clinician had a sinking feeling when entering the room and looking into Mary's eyes—the sparkle wasn't there and her skin looked pale and thin.

Clinician: Mary, it's good to see you. How are you?

Mary: I think I need to sleep more. I'm tired at work, and Mr. Hammon, the new principal at the school where I work, well, he's the one that said I should come see you.

Clinician: I'm glad you're here; let's put our heads together and see if what we come up with. First, let me get a few quick updates. Are you still living by yourself, Mary?

Mary: Yes, just me and that's fine. Well, I do have all of William's stuff in his room, but he's not there. And my grand-daughter, Lucy, she comes to stay sometimes and my daughter, too, sometimes, you know when they have time. How have you been, doctor?

Clinician: I've been well, busy here in the clinic but planning a vacation soon. How about you, Mary, what are you doing for fun? For relaxation?

Mary: Oh, me. Well, I watch movies, the old ones. Sometimes, I eat ice cream.

Clinician: That sounds like a bit of a party, Mary, but then I notice that you are losing weight.

Mary: Oh, yes, that's what the nurse said. I wasn't surprised because my clothes are big on me. I don't have much of an appetite and sometimes forget to eat.

Clinician: Are you still going to church and making those quilts for the preemies?

Mary: No, don't do that anymore. Don't want to.

Clinician: Mary, when you say you don't want to make quilts anymore, how do you feel? Do you feel sad or mad or relieved or what?

Mary: Well, I don't know, I guess mad and sad. It just seems like I don't do that because I'm tired, just worn out and I don't know, it just doesn't matter anymore; someone else can do it.

Clinician: What do you mean, Mary, when you say, "it doesn't matter anymore".

Mary: I don't care about it anymore. My life is a big mess, and I can't seem to fix it.

Clinician: So, your *mind* (pointing to the clinician's head) is saying that there's no way to make things better in your life and that the preemies and church are not priorities right now. I hear that. And I want to slow down for a moment and check in about what your *heart* (pointing to clinician's heart) might have to say about how to make your life fuller, richer in meaning.

Mary: … I don't know; I'm kind of confused and … numb. I don't know what my heart is saying … I am thinking it is aching (beginning to cry).

Clinician: Mary, I know you and I know you are a person who cares a lot and cares deeply. The loss of your son has taken the wind out of your sails.

Mary: Yeah, I don't have any wind and I don't even know if I have sails anymore. I just feel stuck, doctor. After the funeral, I told myself I would go on … go back to work, sort out William's stuff and see if I could give some of it to people who could use it. But now I don't even go in that room. I feel so sad and like no one can understand … I've stopped returning calls from people … and I want the tele, really all the time. I don't even go to my bedroom to sleep. I just doze off in my chair. Except on Sunday when I call to see if I can talk to Lucy; she's my son's daughter, my grand-daughter.

Clinician: So, let's try to figure out this feeling of being "stuck" and see what we can do to get you moving. I'd like to know where we are starting, in terms of how big the problem is. Let's use a scale of 1, it is not a problem, and 10, it is a very big problem. What is it today?

Mary: Mmmm, 10, I'd say 10.

Clinician: Okay, so is it a 10 all the time or sometimes less?

Mary: I think it's less on Sunday before I make the call. I guess that's because I know I've already made my mind up to call, and I'm just keeping my word. I told her after William died that I would always call, that she could count on me.

Clinician: Hmm. That's interesting… the part about making your mind up to do something that's important to you. How do you feel when you make the call?

Mary: Like I'm doing something important. I'm a little scared, like what if she isn't there. But then I tell myself I am keeping my word. And when if she's not there, I feel really lonely. I have the clicker in my hand, so that I can just start clicking through the channels until I find something interesting to watch. That's kind of my life right now, doctor.

Clinician: So, what would you choose, Mary, if you could choose: "Stuck, watching tele, and not feeling" or "Caring, calling, and hurting".

Mary: I'd choose "caring, calling, and hurting" … That's me. I am a person that keeps their word.

Clinician: You are a courageous person, Mary, and I have some ideas about how you might use more of that courage to make your life fuller and to bring more joy into it. First, though, I have to warn you that it is hard to be courageous because it means opening up to your pain—and with William's death, life has dealt you a big one.

Mary: Yes, I guess it has.

In this contextual interview, the clinician experienced a strong emotional response to the patient (i.e., sadness and worry about a rapid decline in physical, mental and social health) and the use of a structured approach to functional assessment helped keep the interview moving toward generation of a precise behavior change plan. Much of the interview was completed at a fast pace, but the pauses (represented by "…" in the clinical dialogues) are intentional and important. The pauses in an interview encourage patients and providers to come into the present moment for more direct experience of avoided thoughts, feelings, and sensations. With greater exposure to difficult thoughts and feelings, more familiarity and acceptance is possible. With more acceptance, the patient's ability to engage in new behaviors, consistent with valued directions, even in the presence of difficult feelings grows.

As with Amy and Bob, the clinician working with Mary helped her define the target problem as they progressed through the problem context questions. While sadness was a problem, it was not the problem that cut Mary off from vitality. The target problem was the class of behaviors Mary described as "being stuck" that blocked her experience of caring. Being stuck robbed her of the energy to strive for connections with the children at her job, participation in her spiritual community, and engagement in charitable activities she had once loved.

Let's take a look at how the contextual interview information can be used to conceptualize an intervention for Mary (See Table 4.10, Mary's Four-Square). The Four-Square analysis helps the clinician understand the impact of being stuck on Mary's life. The lack of feeling is a pervasive theme in her actions that are "not working" and it robs her of energy for engaging in approach activities that are value-consistent (e.g., going to work with an intention to be helpful to the children). In the assessment, the clinician worked to help Mary open to her feelings of loss *and* caring and her sadness may help her break through the numbness.

Let's take a look at what Mary's PAT might look like (See Table 4.11, Mary's PAT). Mary, like many people overwhelmed by loss, has strengths and deficits in all

Table 4.10 Mary's four-square (Example)

	Not Workable	Workable
Actions	Watching TV Staying in the living room at night rather than sleeping in her bed Ignoring phone calls and messages Carefully moving about her home so as to not see William's belongings	Making an appointment to see the clinician Going to work Calling Lucy Talking with Lucy's mother Answering the phone when her daughter calls
Thoughts	It's too late for me. It's not fair. Awful things happen to good people – This is wrong. I should have been able to help William.	Loves her daughter I keep my word. I choose calling, caring, and hurting (sees self as able to hurt in order to show love)
Feelings sensations	Sad Numb	

Table 4.11 Mary's PAT (Example)

Open	Aware	Engaged
• Accepts distressing thoughts and feelings • Creates a safe observational distance from distressing thoughts and feelings • Uses experiences to inform behavior, rather than habits and rules	• Intentionally focuses on present moment experience • Uses self-reflective awareness to promote sensitivity to context • Can change perspectives on stories told about self and others	• Speaks about values with emotion, recalls moments of values-in-action, and accepts vulnerability that comes with caring • Plans and implements behavior change experiments that promote vitality
Strengths	**Strengths**	**Strengths**
Some strengths evidenced by Mary's ability to open to her sadness Tears in the visit Able to hear and use new rule: Choosing caring, calling, and hurting over…	Some strength evidenced by ability to be in the moment in the interview, to be curious about the clinician	Some strength evidenced by connecting caring with hurting; demonstrates ability to show love by continuing to call Lucy
Deficits	**Deficits**	**Deficits**
Lacks skills for opening to grief and sense of vulnerability Unworkable rules: It's done and there's no need to talk about it. I can just shut the door. Numbness	Self-story about "being over" No narrative developed about William and his death **Difficulties connecting with** sensory experience (hunger, etc.)	Difficulties with engaging in value-consistent actions related to William's belongings Little variation in behavior Disconnection from activities that might strengthen value connections (church, quilt group, interaction with children at work)
Targets	**Target**	**Targets**
Assist with detecting and accepting negative and positive feelings Explore feelings in regards to William's death Assist with perspective of compassion for self	Suggest attending to crying, urges to cry and efforts to avoid tears Notice the way she feels after crying (same, better, worse) Take pause breaks from television and notice thoughts and feelings Take pause breaks and engage in sensory experience (drinking cup of tea slowly, sitting outside and looking at anything that's growing)	Encourage interaction with daughter about William's belongings, possibly making some available to those in need Explore possible one-time visit to church, quilting group, church library Suggest she write a brief list of moments that brought her joy when she returns home from work

areas. The clinician has many targets to choose from. Given the extent of Mary's withdrawal from life and from her emotions, it is probably best to focus behavior change planning on activities that wake her up to her feelings and encourage her participation in life. FACT metaphors that support influencing all pillars of flexibility are helpful with people like Mary, and Chap. 5 provides an illustration of the bull's-eye metaphor (Fig. 5.4) to help Mary.

A Note About Suicide and Risk Assessment

Before ending this long section of clinical dialogues and illustration of assessment tools, let's turn our attention to issues related to assessment of suicide and other possible risks (e.g., homicide, interpersonal violence, etc.). Clinicians must be sensitive to possible risks and assess risk when indicated. There are excellent books written on this subject, and readers are encouraged to inform themselves and use evidence-based risk assessment questions in the contextual interview when needed. As this was not our focus, the case illustrations did not include use of risk assessment questions in the contextual interview. The purposes of this chapter and Chap. 5 are to prepare clinicians for completing powerful functional assessments and conceptualizing and implementing precise engaging behavior change plans.

Recommended Strategies for Providing Assessments that Engage Patients in Behavior Change

Table 4.12 provides a Checklist of Recommended Strategies for Using Behavior Change Assessments that Engage Patients. Since it would be difficult to pursue all with equal amounts of attention at the same time, readers need to choose the ones they believe to be of fundamental importance and practice these. Overtime, most readers will be able to integrate all of the strategies into their practice.

1. Prepare the patient to engage in a conversation about behavior change. Use a standard introduction, such as the one provided in this chapter.
2. Use standardized assessments that are brief, acceptable to patients, and clinically useful. Use assessments at all visits to engage patients in evaluating the impact of their behavior change efforts on their quality of life.
3. Understand the patient's current life context, including the impact of the problem on the patient's ability to flourish in key roles, such as being a student, a partner, or a parent. Use the Contextual Assessment Checklist (Table 4.8) to assure that your assessment is complete before you move into active behavior change planning.
4. Understand the context for the presenting problem-the antecedents and the consequences and why change matters at this time. Overtime, use of the Contextual Assessment Questions will shape clinician interviewing skills, so that consideration of the triggers and trajectory of specific behaviors and working with antecedent conditions and consequences becomes routine.
5. Honor a patient's efforts to solve their problem, noting short-term versus long-term usefulness. Patients are problem-solvers, and they often don't see that they are stuck in solutions that are not working. Be curious about their solutions and help them clarify their values.

6. Use assessments in follow-up visits that focus on change in the problem and patient experience with implementing the plan. Patients often show interest in the results of standardized assessments in follow-up visits. A focus on change and patient experience in implementing action plans encourages patient follow through and growth in self-efficacy.

Table 4.12 Checklist: Recommended strategies for using behavior change assessments that engage patients[a]

Selected Strategy	Recommended Strategies
	1. Prepare the patient to engage in a conversation about behavior change.
	2. Use standardized assessments that are brief, acceptable to patients, and clinically useful.
	3. Understand the patient's current life context, including the impact of the problem on the patient's ability to flourish in key roles, such as being a student, a partner, or a parent.
	4. Understand the context for the presenting problem-the antecedents and the consequences and why change matters at this time.
	5. Honor patient's efforts to solve their problem, noting short-term versus long-term usefulness of their solutions.
	6. Use assessments in follow-up visits that focus on change in the problem and patient experience with implementing the plan.

[a]Place a mark beside strategies that you believe would be helpful in your clinic and feasible at this point in time.

Summary

This chapter offered readers a framework for completing assessments that engage patients in behavior change. Assessments begin with a conversation about quality of life and the importance of learning new skills to address problems in living a meaningful life. Focused ACT supports a functional approach to behavior change and helps clinicians identify targets for developing skills that promote psychological flexibility in solving problems. Through case examples and clinical dialogues, readers learned to use the Contextual Interview Questions, the Four Square Tool, and the PAT to assess and conceptualize interventions.

Review

• A standard introduction to assessment informs the patients that the purpose of assessment is to identify factors important to developing a precise and practical plan for behavior change.
• A standardized assessment measure of a patient's health-related quality of life is useful at initial and follow-up visits.

- The Contextual Assessment Questions (Table 4.1) help clinicians complete time-effective functional assessments.
- The Four-Square Tool (Table 4.2) helps clinicians understand the function of behaviors identified in a contextual assessment.
- The FACT Pillars Assessment Tool encourages (Table 4.3) further understanding of a patient's strengths and weaknesses in three areas of psychological flexibility: openness, awareness, and engagement.
- Use the Checklist of Recommended Strategies for Assessments that Promote Behavior Change (Table 4.12) to select a few initial targets and discuss these with clinic leaders. Also, share the Tips for Leaders table (Table 4.13).

Table 4.13 Tips for leaders

1. In the Electronic Health Record (EHR), assist with building smart phrases to create reminder lists for key assessment questions (e.g., Contextual Interview questions), as this will support consistency among team members and time-effective interviewing.
2. Integrate visit rating scores, such as the problem severity rating, into the EHR, as these are useful clinically and in monthly reports for clinicians to use in evaluating their services.
3. Create aggregate data fields in the EHR for standardized behavioral health measures, such as health-related quality of life scores.
4. Create reports using behavioral health measures to help the team better understand their patients and the impact of their services.

References

American Psychiatric Association. (2016). *Diagnostic and statistical manual of mental disorders* (5th ed.. (DSM-5)). Washington, D. C: American Psychological Association.

Bond, F. W., Hayes, S. C., Baer, R. A., Carpenter, K. M., Guenole, N., Orcutt, H. K., … Zettle, R. D. (2011). Preliminary psychometric properties of the acceptance and action questionnaire – II: A revised measure of psychological inflexibility and experiential avoidance. *Behavior Therapy, 42*(4), 676–688. https://doi.org/10.1016/j.beth.2011.03.007

Duke Family Medicine and Community Health Department. Duke Health Profile (DUKE), Duke Health Profile-8 (Duke-8) and the Duke Population Health Profile (Duke-PH, for details see https://fmch.duke.edu/research/duke-health-measures).

Frances, A. (2012) Two fallacies invalidate the DSM-5 field trials. Psychiatric times, January 10, 2012. https://www.psychiatrictimes.com/dsm-5/two-fallacies-invalidate-dsm-5-field-trials Accessed 20 July 2019.

Hayes, S. C., Strosahl, K. D., & Wilson, K. G. (2012). Acceptance and commitment therapy. In *The process and practice of mindful change* (2nd ed.). New York, NY: Guilford.

Robinson, P., Gould, D., & Strosahl, K. (2010). *Real behavior change in primary care: Improving outcomes and increasing job satisfaction*. Oakland, CA: New Harbinger.

Strosahl, K., Robinson, P., & Gustavsson, T. (2012). *Brief interventions for radical change: Focused acceptance and commitment therapy*. Oakland, CA: New Harbinger.

Chapter 5
Behavior Change in Primary Care: Interventions

Abbreviations

BHC	Behavioral health clinician
BMI	Body Mass Index
CBS	Contextual Behavioral Science (Scientist)
CBSC	Contextual Behavioral Scientist Check-in
CBT	Cognitive Behavioral Therapy
CBT-I	Cognitive Behavioral Therapy-Insomnia
CHW	Community health worker
EHR	Electric Health Record
FACT	Focused Acceptance and Commitment Therapy
HC	Health Coach
PIG	Pillar Intervention Guide
PAT	Pillar Assessment Tool
PC	Primary Care
PCBH	Primary Care Behavioral Health model
PCC	Primary Care Clinician
PT	Physical Therapist
PTSD	Post-Traumatic Stress Disorder

This chapter provides practical guidance on using a contextual approach to improve behavioral health outcomes at the population level. Readers will learn about *Primary Care Behavioral Health* (PCBH) strategies and their importance in defining the qualities for a delivery platform, a "syringe" capable of holding powerful medicines for behavior change. Amy, Bob, and Mary (introduced in Chap. 4) return in clinician-patient dialogues, offering opportunities for demonstration of the use of the *Pillars Intervention Guide* to increase psychological flexibility. The chapter offers a variety of worksheets for readers to use in clinical practice, including one for engaging patients in meaningful conversations about values and another for creating powerful behavioral experiments. The chapter also provides a *Contextual Behavioral*

© The Author(s), under exclusive license to Springer Nature
Switzerland AG Pte Ltd 2019
P. J. Robinson, *Basics of Behavior Change in Primary Care*, SpringerBriefs
in Psychology, https://doi.org/10.1007/978-3-030-32050-8_5

Scientist Check-In for readers to use now and over time to assess their progress in delivering powerful behavior change interventions. This is the last chapter of the book and it concludes with the usual checklist of strategies for readers to use in setting priorities.

A Syringe and Powerful Medicines

A population-based care approach to behavior change requires that a clinician have both a powerful syringe and power medicines for behavior change. The success of one depends upon the success of the other. However, without the syringe, fewer people with receive the medicine. Key syringe features include accessibility, brevity, team-based care, and ease of deployment. Medicines need to have an evidenced base and be easily mastered by a diverse group of clinicians with differing levels of training in behavioral science.

Primary Care Behavioral Health

The *Primary Care Behavioral Health* (PCBH) model describes a team-focused approach to delivery of behavioral health interventions in PC, and its strategies are useful in describing the key components of a platform for behavior change or an effective syringe. The model was extensively detailed by Robinson and Reiter (2007, 2015) and was the focus of a recent special edition of the *Journal of Clinical Psychology in Medical Settings* (Reiter, Dobmeyer & Hunter, 2017). A recent review of 29 studies on the PCBH model found that it shows promise as an effective population health approach to behavioral health service delivery and that it is associated with positive patient and implementation outcomes (Hunter, Funderburk, Polaha, Bauman, Goodie, & Hunter, 2017a).

The model suggests addition of a mental health provider to the primary care (PC) team (i.e., a *Behavioral Health Consultant*, BHC). Some clinics will hire multiple BHCs, while other clinics, due to insufficient resources, may need to collaborate with BHCs located externally from their clinics. Internally or externally located, the role of the BHC is to support team efforts to provide effective behavioral health interventions. The work of internal BHCs mirrors that of *Primary Care Clinicians* (PCCs) and nurses. It is accessible, continuous, and coordinated. BHC chart notes are considered as PC notes and entered into the medical record. PCCs and nursing staff can easily see, support and eventually independently implement many interventions started in BHC visits. Evidence-based behavioral, cognitive, and motivational interviewing interventions are strong medicines, whether delivered by a BHC or other clinicians working in PC.

The design and delivery of BHC services are influenced by two over-arching goals. The first goal is to help patients learn be more effective in promoting their biological, psychological and social health. The second goal is to help PCCs, nursing staff, *Physical Therapist* (PTs), *Health Coaches* (HCs) and others doing behavior change work in PC learn to implement effective biopsychosocial assessments and interventions.

The PCBH approach provides a strong foundation for addressing behavior change opportunities, including those with a preventive, acute care, and chronic care focus. By helping patients learn skills to prevent illness, healthcare dollars are generated for services designed to reduce health disparities (i.e., the negative health status differences between an identified subgroup in comparison with other sub-groups or the population as a whole). The PCBH approach will help PC attain improvements for health at the population level, where all experience better health outcomes (Starfield, Shi, & Macinko, 2005). PCBH methods are also useful for informing integration activities for other new PC team members, such as pharmacists (see Gallimore, Corso, Robinson, & Runyan, 2018).

Powerful Medicines

Cognitive Behavioral Therapy (CBT) and *Focused Acceptance and Commitment Therapy* (FACT) are powerful medicines for clinicians working to improve health outcomes for PC patients. Dr. Dobmeyer's book, *Psychological Treatment of Medical Patients in Integrated Primary Care*, provides instructions on using CBT with patients experiencing depression, anxiety, insomnia, diabetes, chronic pain, and asthma (Dobmeyer, 2018). There are other excellent resources for readers to study to learn more about using CBT in PC behavior change visits (see for example, Hunter, Goodie, Oordt, & Dobmeyer, 2017b). There are a variety of CBT-informed patient education materials for children, youth and adults on this book's website (basicsofbehaviorchangeinprimarycare.com). Research documenting the effectiveness of CBT interventions in brief PC visits for conditions such as insomnia (Goodie, Isler, Hunter, & Peterson, 2009) and post-traumatic stress disorder (PTSD, Cigrang, Rauch, Avila, Bryan, Goodie, Hryshko-Mullen, Peterson, 2011) is growing, with a number of studies in progress at this time.

Focused Acceptance and Commitment Therapy

Focused Acceptance and Commitment Therapy (FACT) is ideal for PC because it is by design intended for brief visits and team-based support of behavior change. Several books provide detailed information on using FACT to guide brief assessments and deliver brief interventions (see Robinson, Gould & Strosahl, 2010 and Strosahl, Robinson & Gould, 2012). In FACT, the clinician focuses on helping the patient improve their functioning and frames symptoms as important and useful, as they relate to what the patient cares about. The FACT approach is less focused on diagnostic interviewing and more focused on promoting psychological flexibility.

It is useful in individual, couple, family and group interventions. The *Life Path* and *Bull's-eye* metaphors presented later in this chapter can be used in groups as well as individual visits. Results from a study of a 4-week FACT Life Path class found large improvements in quality of life (Glover, et al., 2016). The manual for this class is available on this book's website (basicsofbehaviorchangeinprimarycare.com).

Generating Information to Inform Interventions for Primary Care

Historically, researchers have attempted to answer the question, "Which treatment works best for which problem?" With a lack of attention to contextual factors, such as treatment setting, patient motivation and preparation of clinicians, behavior change clinicians have had to adapt treatments to fit the PC context. Delivery of evidence-based interventions sized for PC has been found to improve patient's use of targeted skills 6 months after completing the intervention (Robinson, VonKorff, Bush, Ludman, & Lin, 2020), suggesting that the adaptation approach is workable. The Coping Strategies Use Scale (Robinson, Von Korf, Bush, Linn, & Ludman, 2020), measures rates of use of behavioral strategies and is an alternative to symptom rating screeners (see this book's website: basicsofbehaviorchangeinprimary-care.com).

A more expeditious approach to development of population-based behavioral interventions is possible when researchers ask different questions. Strosahl and Robinson recommend the following.

> Which treatment(s) works best, in the shortest possible time, with the least resources used, with the lowest refusal and attrition rates, when delivered by mental health and non–mental-health providers (with different levels of training) in a variety of different community settings, and with patients suffering from medical and mental health conditions of varying levels of severity? (Strosahl & Robinson, 2018, p. 8).

Over the next decade, more researchers will investigate interventions with the idea of population impact in mind. Their studies will help inform interventions for PC and enhance health outcomes. For now, this chapter offers readers an opportunity to learn a contextual approach to behavior change, FACT, and when used in the powerful syringe of PCBH, it is likely to support better health outcomes at the population level.

Promoting Psychological Flexibility in Clinical Contacts

Focused Acceptance and Commitment Therapy works well in short visits, is engaging for patients, helps patients with varying levels of severity, and can be delivered by non-mental health and mental health providers. The goal of FACT is to help patients develop skills to solve problems of living more successfully. The group of skills center around the general characteristic of psychological flexibility, contrasted with psychological inflexibility (where a patient continues with the same behaviors that are not serving their interests). When a person is psychologically flexible, they are able to be present in the moment, to understand available options, and to pursue a course of action consistent with their freely chosen values. With higher levels of flexibility, a person is able to accept and fully experience emotional pain that comes into their lives, whatever the source. They are also more able to be present and to learn from the direct consequences of their behavior. While thoughts, emotions, and sensations are sometimes helpful, they are not always useful guides for long-term choices. Thoughts, feelings, and sensations come and go, while our values or principles for living are stable anchors for decision-making and for charting a course of action.

Focused Acceptance and Commitment Therapy identifies Three Pillars of Psychological Flexibility: Open, Aware, and Engaged. The *FACT Pillars Assessment Tool* (PAT, Fig. 4.1), introduced in Chap. 4, provides descriptions of behavioral qualities demonstrated by individuals with greater psychological flexibility in each of the three pillars: Open, Aware and Engaged.

As mentioned previously, a person's ability to be open, aware and engaged may change when the person's life context changes. For example, most people experience a loss in flexibility with an increase in life stress, such as losing a loved one or being the victim of interpersonal violence. Chapter 4 provided examples of using the FACT Pillars Assessment Tool (PAT, Table 4.9) to gauge a patient's psychological flexibility and set pillar targets.

The FACT Pillars Intervention Guide

The FACT Pillars Intervention Guide (PIG, Table 5.1) provides suggestions for clinicians concerning targeting specific pillars. Clinicians may be able to assess a patient's level of psychological flexibility and target one or more specific pillars

Table 5.1 FACT Pillar Intervention Guide (PIG)

When intervening with patients, use the suggested guides to assist with moment-to-moment interactions that move the patient toward greater psychological flexibility

Open	Aware	Engaged
When "stuck", be curious, model acceptance, notice the "mind"	If confused, go to the present, look at different perspectives	Whenever possible, promote connection between values and action
Support openness and curiosity about previously avoided thoughts/ feelings/ sensations	**Promote flexible, voluntary and purposeful attention to the present moment**	Identify qualities of meaningful action in the here and now
Attend to thinking as an ongoing process, rather than the world structured by it	Support mindfulness and noticing of the continuity of consciousness	Collaboratively create SMART behavioral experiments

intentionally during a visit to benefit the patient's overall functioning. Let's look at the guides for each of the pillars.

Open

The PIG suggests that clinicians adopt an attitude of curiosity when patients appear to be stuck, doing the same behaviors again and again or following the same unquestioned rules without awareness. The clinician might suggest that the patient experiment with a new observational distance from a rule, thought, memory or emotion by simply moving toward a perspective of noticing. To help the patient, the clinician might alternatively suggest that the patient use a description to frame the experience, such as "I am having the thought that I'm all messed up" or "I am having the feeling called sad."

To help the patient open more to avoided experiences, the clinician might ask the patient to stay with the difficult thought or feeling, opening to it and letting it be there. Useful questions when targeting openness include, "So your mind is telling you ..." and "What does the human choose at this moment?"

As patients open to avoided experiences, they begin to see that thinking is an on-going process, sometimes useful and sometimes not. Thinking or feeling does not have to structure perception of the world; there are other levels of observation that allow patients much more freedom to choose behaviors consistent with what is most important to them. In a later part of this section, the interaction between a clinician and Amy, the 15-year-old brought to the clinic by her mother in Chap. 4, illustrate targeting the *Open* and *Aware* pillars to enhance psychological flexibility.

Aware

While the conversation that supports behavior change in the moment sometimes flows, it may get stuck with the patient repeating a story or providing unnecessary details about an old narrative. The clinician often senses that nothing is really happening and may be confused about how to change the interaction to make it better support in-the-moment change. The patient may be telling a story because they are on "automatic", and the clinician is just sitting back and listening because they don't know what to do. These are signals of lack of awareness and the lack of awareness can interfere with change in the both the *Open* and *Engaged* pillars of psychological flexibility. The clinician might ask the patient to tune into their breath, just noticing if it is shallow or deep, slow or fast. The clinician could ask the patient to notice what's happening in their head—the pace of their thinking. Alternatively, they might suggest the importance of taking stock of what is happening in the body (i.e., the level of tension or heaviness). In the realm of emotional experience, is there an emotional tone operating beyond awareness? If the patient is telling a story about themselves or others or both, what is the quality of the story. Is it new or old? Is it told self-reflectively or automatically?

Values

The FACT PIG advises clinicians to pursue values clarification and develop a behavioral experiment informed by the patient's values *whenever the opportunity arises*. An opportunity arises whenever patients talk about what or who is important relative to the problem they are facing. For example, a patient with symptoms of depression and anxiety might say, "I want to do something about this because my 20- and 22-year old daughters are watching and I want them to see that I'm trying to better myself, even though I have a lot of problems. If they see I'm trying, they'll know that it's important to keep trying and then I'm hoping that they'll be able to make their lives better than mine." This statement provides the clinician with an opportunity to take the conversation in a direction that promotes an even stronger connection with patient values and perhaps to teach skills that would promote persistence in experimenting with new behaviors.

Targeting Open and Aware

The case example of Amy provides an opportunity to look at how a clinician can follow the PIG recommendations for targeting *Open* and *Aware* pillars to promote greater flexibility in a clinic visit. As you will recall from Chap. 4, information from *Contextual Interview Questions* (Table 4.1) led the clinician and Amy to identify a target problem of "feeling sick inside" and leaving school without permission. The Four-Square analysis identified a long list of difficult thoughts, feelings, and sensations that Amy wanted to avoid (See Table 4.2). At the same time, Amy has many strengths that could buffer the impact of the many adversities that had happened in her young life. She is at a critical moment in her life, where she could easily become stuck in actions that help her avoid very painful inner experiences and bring worse health outcomes, namely that of using alcohol and tobacco.

Using the *Pillars Assessment Tool* (PAT, Table 4.3) and the *Four-Square Tool* (Table 4.6), the clinician understood the high stakes of caring for Amy at a vulnerable time and in close proximity to an assumed tragic and painful violent experience. The clinician wanted to pace interventions with Amy and decided that shoring up her strengths and helping her build out her skills for coping independently was a priority. Amy's life circumstance was pulling her toward adulthood at a pace that the clinician wanted to slow down but could not. By helping her build out her skills for coping effectively, the clinician hoped to encourage Amy's trust and enhance the possibilities for future visits to clarify, re-shape and add onto painful internal experiences that could block her progress toward goals of going to college and having an interesting career. The clinician hoped to target *Open* and *Aware* pillars in order to help her make gains in psychological flexibility.

Amy: Thanks. It's nice to know that you care and that you're not going to rat on me to my Mom. She has a really hard life, and she can get really mad ... scary mad.

Clinician: You know, Amy, I think you have a pretty hard life, too, and I think you are one heck-of-a-strong person. I want us to work on a couple of little routines in your life that may help you stay on track with school and your brother and with going to college, too. First, I want us to figure out how you can be a bit of a detective and catch that "sick inside" feeling when it first starts to happen. What do you know about that? What do you feel first? Does it happen any particular place in your body?

Amy: I don't like to think about it but I will if you think it will help me...

Clinician: Maybe for a few minutes we could explore it together, just to see what it is and where it happens.

Amy: I think maybe I feel sick in my chest, my heart first-here (pointing to her chest); kind of like there's something heavy on top of me and it's like I can't breathe. From there, my head just fills up and I start crying and walking or running. That's all I want to feel right now, okay.

Clinician: Got it, so let's just take a deep breath and thank those feelings and sensations for showing up so we could get a new perspective on them—one with a nice distance, huh? Maybe you could bring your little brother's face to mind; you had such a soft expression when you spoke of him a few minutes ago.

Amy: Okay. You know, Sam is pretty special. He's a really good person.

Clinician: So, this is what I'm thinking. I want you to try to breathe out as much air as you can and then even a little more ... (demonstrating) ... and then (demonstrating) breathe in slowly and pause. Go ahead and try it again, breathe out, yes, all the way, and then it's easy to breathe in. Two more times now, very slow breaths. How's that?

Amy: Better. I feel better. Is that what you want me to do? Breathe out three times when I feel that pressure in my chest.

Clinician: Yes, and let's add a few more things. Let's try having you put your hand on your heart and silently say something kind to yourself, like "You are safe now. You are loved. You are a sweet big sister". You'll need to find your own words. What are your ideas?

Amy: I like the sweet big sister. That makes me feel calmer. I tell my brother that he is my sweet boy and that I love him when I put him to bed at night.

Clinician: Very nice, Amy. I like that. And the second routine that I wanted to talk about was for the evening hours with your brother. I'd like to see if we can help you sleep better, and there's a couple of things that might help. First, I think it's important that you and your brother get lots of physical activity after school—

walking, dance or exercise videos, anything that uses up your energy. Second, I think it's important that you have a routine for a couple of hours before sleep that helps you relax. During those two hours, you can do things like finish homework, but then turn off all screens and take a bath or shower, read, listen to calm music, maybe even do some kid yoga with your brother—the relaxing kind. We want a routine that helps you prepare for sleep.

Amy: Well, I like those ideas. That would be really different from what I've been doing recently. I usually read with Sam and then put him to bed. Then, I get up and watch crime shows while I play games on my phone and do homework. A change in routines could help.

Clinician: Do you sleep in the same room as your brother?

Amy: Yes, we sleep in the same bed ... Mom is going to get us twin beds when we get enough money. I don't mind sleeping with him; he doesn't move around that much.

Clinician: Well, maybe you could try tucking in with him and see if you fall asleep. If you don't, you could always get up and do some stretching or read your most boring school book – just use low light and have the light coming from behind you so that it is not too bright. Bright light tends to wake us up.

Amy: I didn't know that.

In this brief exchange, the clinician targets Amy's openness to her troubling thoughts, feelings, and sensations and helps her develop a new relationship with them. The suggested routine allows her to recognize her need for a sense of safety and to create that for herself by slowing down (breathing in a way that stimulates her parasympathetic nervous system) and using an image of her younger brother to evoke sensations of nurturing and love. In order to make this gain in psychological flexibility, Amy used skills related to the *Awareness* pillar, namely the ability to tune in to sensations. Using *Open* and *Aware* together helped create an in-clinic change in behavior that Amy can use outside the clinic in her day-to-day life.

Targeting Values

The clinician working with Bob in Chap. 4 was concerned about Bob's reluctance to use PC for his medical problems and wanted to pursue an intervention that would encourage engagement in the future. The Four-Square analysis of Bob's contextual interview information suggested a somewhat short list of workable actions and a long list of unworkable thoughts, feelings, and sensations, along with some easy to execute avoidance behaviors (i.e., beer and television). Bob's thoughts and feelings about the importance of family and health were strengths the clinician could use to encourage more value consistent actions.

Table 5.2 The "Relate the Problem to Values" worksheet

Experiment with using one or more of these questions to assist the patient with seeing a relationship between the problem and values that are important to the patient at this time.

1. Tell me more about why it is important for you to find a new way to address this problem now.

2. In a world where anything is possible, what would you do about this problem?

3. If you could make this problem go away, but it cost you the ability to care about problems like this, would you?

4. If you didn't have x as value, would this problem matter to you?

5. What does your heart say about this problem?

6. What happens in your body now when we are talking about this?

Consider patient answers to questions asked and conceptualize a plan that would be important to the patient.

Are there skills that you could teach the patient during the visit to strengthen the patient's ability to implement the plan?

The "Relate the Problem to Values" Worksheet

The clinician had recently studied the *Relate the Problem to Values Worksheet* (Table 5.2) and used it to inspire his work with Bob, as demonstrated in the following dialogue. This worksheet encourages the clinician to explore the relationship between the problem and the patient's values and to go beyond any narrow view on the problem to a perspective of possibility. Often, clinicians are more successful in targeting values if they simultaneously target *Awareness*. The clinician's interaction with Bob demonstrates the power of this combination.

Clinician: Bob, I'd like to know a little more about the kinds of things you do or could do outside of work to counter-balance the stress of work. Like, what sorts of fun activities or hobbies might appeal to you at this point.

Bob: I don't know. I just seem to be out-of-gas after work and want to go straight home. I used to hit a bucket of balls sometimes on the way home, but not in a while.

Clinician: Okay, that's a possibility. What else might you do? Maybe something with your wife or your son or a friend.

Bob: Well, my son and I used to watch a game together – you know like be on the phone with each other during the Sunday game. I've stopped doing that. A little embarrassed to say that I worry about his thinking that I'm drinking too much. He's like his mother; all uptight about me having a little beer.

Clinician: I see. Well, let's keep watching a game with your son as a possibility. How about your wife, any possibilities of doing something with her?

Bob: Well, my wife and I had a Five Dollar Tuesday movie date for a while but I've been dodging that, really for the same reason – just easier to sit on the couch and watch sports, lots on right now.

Clinician: Do you like going to movies with your wife?

Bob: Well, yeah, it's okay after we get there. I guess I kind of do. I like that she likes it, too, if you know what I mean.

Clinician: Sure, I understand. You feel happy when you see her happy.

Bob: Yep. And I don't think she's very happy with me lately.

Clinician: Okay, movies are on the list. Now, let's see … Is there any possible stress-relieving activity that is physical?

Bob: I used to walk down to the park at lunch sometimes, but I stopped when the new manager arrived. Guess I could try that; it does kind of wake me up and settle me down at the same time—you know just getting out of the store.

Clinician: Did the walk or being in the park give you a feeling of peace and calm?

Bob: Yes, I guess so. Same as hitting a bucket of balls, gives my mind something to focus on.

Clinician: So, I've made a list of possibilities for balancing work stress. One: Watch Sunday game with your son. Two: Tuesday movie night with your wife. Three: Walking to the park at lunch. Four: Hitting a bucket of balls on the way home.

Bob: That's a nice list doctor.

Clinician: Yes, I think so and I think it might just be a list … so how about we take a moment to look at why it's important for you to do something different in dealing with the stressful situation at work.

Bob: We'll, so I can get my wife off my back and not have to take those happy pills I guess (smiling).

Clinician: Right, I get that. But seriously, Bob, what matters and who matters in this situation.

Bob: Well, I do matter. I've gained more weight and I feel tired a lot more of the time, so I need to do something different for me.

Clinician: Who else matters?

Bob: Hmmm. Well, of course my son and wife. I want them to respect me and believe in me. Both of them have said I am drinking a lot of beer these days – I used to only drink on weekends. I don't want them to lose respect for me … (looking down). My Dad was a big beer drinker, and I told myself I'd never be like him. Don't get me wrong, I loved him and he wasn't a mean drunk or anything, just kind of stupid and then sometimes things would get out of control and he'd end up vomiting in the bathroom. I kind of pitied him but I think I also kind of hated him sometimes … you know for losing control.

Clinician: Bob, you are worthy of respect, respect from your son, wife, and yourself and pursuing respect is a good reason to try some new behaviors. Sounds like you also want them to see you as a good problem solver, and I think that is also an important consideration in deciding how to address your problem at work.

Bob: Yeah, that's right. Respect and problem solving are important to me.

Clinician: And that's why you care about the problem at work. What does your heart say that you should do at this point?

Bob: Well, be stronger at work and try to help the new manager more. And do more for the people I care about – like the things you have on the list—Sunday games with my son and Tuesday movies with my wife.

The quality of the interactions leading to a plan for a behavioral experiment improved with the clinician's use of a few questions from the *Relate the Problem to the Values Worksheet* (Table 5.2). With only a few minutes more of conversation, Bob made a connection with his past relationship with his father and the ways he wanted to relate to important people in his life now. That connection helped him take ownership of an evolving plan that only minutes before had been "just a list".

Behavioral Experiments

A *behavioral experiment* is a plan that identifies one or more specific actions a patient plans to take in order to impact the problem of concern in a more meaningful way. It may be an observable action that the patient plans to take with others or alone, in their homes, a work context or the community. It may be an action that involves working with difficult thoughts and feelings in a new way, such as a 5-minute practice of sitting still and noticing thoughts and feelings with an attitude of curiosity. Clinicians often ask, "What is good behavioral experiment?"

The bottom-line answer is a good experiment is one that the patient will do and will learn from. If the patient doesn't implement the experiment after the contact and is also unable to identify on barriers that interfered, then the possibility of meaningful change doesn't move forward. The goal of a behavioral experiment is always *behavioral variability*. In this section, readers will learn about variability, use the *SMART Behavioral Experiment Worksheet* (Table 5.3), and read clinician patient-dialogues illustrating development of behavioral experiments with Bob and Amy.

Behavioral Variability

Behavioral variability simply means doing something new and different and noticing what happens. Promoting behavioral variability requires the clinician to attend to three factors. First, the clinician must assure that patients understand the purpose of experimenting. Second, the clinician needs to assure that patients are confident in the plan before ending the visit. Third, the clinician needs to create a values context for the plan and assure that the plan is in some way related to the patient's values as they pertain to the problem of concern. Let's look at each of these three factors.

Table 5.3 The "SMART Behavioral Experiment" worksheet

Use this worksheet to improve your skills for developing behavioral experiments with patients. If the patient's history included painful punishing experiences (e.g., critical or depressed parent, multiple traumas), you may want to spend a little more time explaining the value of experimenting and the usefulness of trying something new.

A SMART behavioral experiment is engaging and SMART*

A. Is the experiment engaging?

   1. What does "experimenting" mean to the patient?

   2. Can the patient imagine doing the experiment?

   3. Is there any part of the experiment that the patient may need to practice with the clinician before the end of the visit?

   4. What might get in the way of the patient *doing* the experiment?

   5. Is the patient confident about *doing* the experiment? 1 is not at all confident and 10 is very confident

If not a 7 or higher in confidence ask, "How shall we change this to bring up your confidence?"

B. Is the experiment SMART?

   ☐ Specific

   ☐ Measurable

   ☐ Attainable

   ☐ Relevant to patient's values

   ☐ Timely

* Inspired by YourCoach, BVBA;https://www.yourcoach.be/en/coaching-tools/smart-goal-

The purpose of experimenting behaviorally is to do something different and see what happens, and that includes what happens *inside the person and outside the person*. Patients benefit from clear instructions about being aware while they conduct an experiment, much like a scientist who attends to all the factors potentially influencing a laboratory experiment. Patients need to attend to what happens immediately preceding, during and immediately after engaging in an experiment. Only with attention to the experiment can the patient fully learn what is there to be learned from the experiment and use this information to inform future experiments. In repeating the process of experimenting and learning, patients may engage in ever-widening circles of variable behavior. The behavioral experiment is the patient's way out of *being stuck* (i.e., engaging in old habits and automatic behaviors that constrain their ability to flourish).

In explaining the purpose of the experiment, clinicians may suggest that, "Failure is useful" in experimenting. This may be particularly important for patients who have learned from authority figures who were highly critical and discouraged their exploration; to engage in experiments these patients may need reassurance about the usefulness of failing and benefit from a discussion of *failing mindfully*. Failing to do the experiment is not a problem if having the plan helped the patient identify the barriers to implementation. Failure of the experiment to change the problem is awesome because the clinician and patient then know what not to do more of (or sometimes, how to change the plan slightly or better prepare the patient so that the plan is more do-able). When we fail mindfully, we learn, and failing mindfully can be even more useful at times than succeeding mindfully.

Confidence

The second factor related to promoting behavioral variability through planned experiments concerns the patient's level of confidence in the plan. Chapter 4, I introduced use of a rating scale to assess the level of confidence a patient has in a plan. The question is asked as soon as the plan has been written, either by the patient or the clinician. Pointing at the written plan, the clinician asks the patient, "On a scale of one to ten, how confident are you in the plan, with one meaning that you are not going to *do* the plan and ten meaning that you are very confident – you will *do* the plan?"

It is recommended that the plan be recorded before the clinician asks the confidence question. Writing the plan and reviewing the written plan provides a stronger level of mutual agreement about what the plan entails. The clinician aims to have patients give confidence ratings of seven or above. If below seven, the clinician needs to ask the patient, "How can we change this plan to get your confidence to a seven?"

Patients can usually suggest modifications and then modifications can be made to the written plan to reflect the details of the final experiment.

A variety of factors may affect the patient's level of confidence, including the resources and skills the patient has available for implementing the plan. When a patient has social support for a plan, they are likely to feel more confident than when they do not. Social support is an important resource when patients aim to engage in a new behavior. When it is not available, the clinician may offer additional support, such as a brief phone call to the patient to inquire about patient experience with the plan several days after the visit. Other resources may be important to consider, depending on the plan. For example, a plan involving eating a better breakfast may be influenced by the patient's resources for obtaining healthy foods.

Patient skills also play an important role in their confidence about implementing a behavioral experiment. Often, clinicians as well as patients may not anticipate the pre-requisite skills needed for a patient to implement a plan. It is not unusual for a patient to voice enthusiasm for engaging in a plan that involves an important inter-personal interaction during the interview and then voice low confidence in the plan. Experiments involving interpersonal behavior changes may require a variety of foundation skills.

For example, a patient might agree to make an appointment to discuss work con-ditions with a manager that seems to have unrealistic expectations for their perfor-mance and then provide a low confidence rating. In exploring the lack of confidence, both clinician and patient may quickly identify the need for prerequisite skill train-ing such as knowledge about the difference between aggressive and passive behav-ior and the option of an assertive statement. The clinician can provide brief instructions and help formulate a plan that has the patient practicing an assertive request in a context that builds skill, such as with a supportive partner or even in the bathroom mirror, prior to talking with the manager. The confidence question is very useful for identifying barriers to implementation of the plan and formulating new plans that better address the barriers and build toward variability.

Values

When patients connect with their values and see the relationship between their val-ues and the problem, they move toward behavior change with greater capacity for commitment. For this reason, it is always a good idea to create a values context when designing behavior change interventions. As readers may recall from Chap. 4, the *Contextual Interview Questions (Table 4.1),* include a question about workability. The workability question moves the interview toward a discussion of values and how they relate to solving the problem the patient is facing. The *Relate the Problem to Values Worksheet* (Table 5.2) offers guidance for discussions about values, their relationship to the problem, and the formulation of a behavioral experiment. As a part of the confidence assessment, clinicians may add a question to check on the relationship between the experiment and the plan, "Does our plan reflect what mat-ters and who matters to you at this moment?"

Engaging in new behavior is challenging. A focus on the importance of change helps the patient dignify the level of discomfort they may feel in implementing an important and difficult behavioral experiment.

A Note about Time and Behavioral Experiments

In addition to three important foundations for creating behavioral experiments that promote behavioral variability, time is a huge factor for clinicians practicing in the busy context of PC. Clinicians might use the perspective of a baseball player to identify the range of options for behavior change when time is limited. If a clinician only has less than 10 minutes with a patient, the visit still needs to include development of a behavioral experiment. Of course, a behavior change plan developed in a 7-minute visit may look different from one cultivated in a 20-minute where the clinician has been able to assess and influence the patient's psychological flexibility. Let's take a look at the differences between a single, a double, a triple, a home run, and a grand slam.

When a clinician has less than 10 minutes to promote behavior change, the aim is a single or a double. In a single or double, the clinician will attempt to understand the context of the problem (including the importance of making a change at this time) and then suggest one or more ideas for change. The clinician will go with the patient's choice and shape it so that it is specific, measurable, and feasible; write it down for the patient to take with them, and, then, ask the patient to rate their confidence in the plan. The difference between a single and a double is having one or two aspects to the plan. One is a single and a single is always sufficient if the patient has confidence in the plan. A double is great, but only if it is feasible for the patient. As a general rule, clinicians can go for a double when the patient seems motivated and there are two actions that are likely to move the patient forward (e.g., eating a small breakfast and taking a 15 minute walk in the park after work). If the patient rates confidence in a double lower than seven, the clinician can move the plan to a single by asking the patient to choose the part of the plan that is most feasible and important.

When the clinician has 10–15 minutes and knows the patient, a triple behavioral experiment is possible. A triple involves design of a behavioral experiment that requires the patient to engage in a behavioral experiment that require more risk-taking (e.g., initiating a conversation concerning how to improve a relationship that is not going well). Many behavioral experiments that involve engaging in an interpersonal behavior may require prerequisite skill training or at least a brief practice between the clinician and the patient.

For example, a clinician might see a patient known to them about a family problem. In a 15-minute visit, the clinician might help the patient develop a behavioral experiment involving interacting with one of their family members in a new way. In order to get to a triple, the clinician would take the time to anticipate what the patient would say, assess the patient's skill in saying it by suggesting a brief practice during the visit, and, then, provide needed coaching or instruction to enhance the likelihood of patient success.

Homeruns can happen anytime, but they probably happen more often when the clinician and patient have time to work through a complete contextual assessment and intervention. This process most commonly requires 20–25 minutes (including charting the note associated with the visit). With homeruns, the clinician is able to create change in the context of the visit, positively influencing the patient's level of psychological flexibility and then formulate a behavioral experiment that promotes practice of skills associated with greater psychological flexibility after the visit in the context of the patient's home, work or community.

Singles are great; doubles and triples are great; homeruns are great. The most important thing in promoting behavior change is to use the time available. Clinicians need not back away from promoting behavioral variability because of time. Patients come to PC looking for help, and clinicians have lots to offer. With continued use of the tools provided in this book, readers will gain skill and efficiency in promoting behavior changes that help their patients flourish.

The SMART Behavioral Experiment Worksheet The *SMART Behavioral Experiment Worksheet* (Table 5.3) offers guidance on how to develop behavioral experiments that are engaging for patients, precise, important, and feasible. The first section offers clinicians a list of questions that are helpful in engaging patients in a conversation about change. Many of these questions were used in the previous section and readers will see some illustrated in the interaction between Mary and Bob in the following section.

The second section of this worksheet is an adaptation of a well-known acronym: SMART   (https://www.yourcoach.be/en/coaching-tools/smart-goal-setting.php). The worksheet invites clinicians to evaluate the quality of their behavioral experiment from the perspective of goal-setting. While values are global, abstract, and not attainable, goals are specific, concrete, and, if planned well, attainable. This section of the checklist asks the clinician to check the quality of the behavioral experiment. There are five criteria: is the experiment or plan specific, measurable, attainable, relevant to the patient's values, and timely? A plan that is specific includes details about what the patient will do, when, and how often. A measurable plan includes an assessment strategy (e.g., the number of times the patient will do the planned activity, the minutes the patient plans to spend eating the dinner meal, etc.). Measurement helps the patient see to see the extent to which they engaged in the planned experiment. Simply counting a target behavior is a useful tool for modifying behavior. Self-monitoring (the formal name for tracking the occurrence of a behavior) is associated with reducing behaviors a patient wants to reduce (e.g., number of cigarettes smoked, bottles of beer consumed, hours spent playing video games) and with increasing behaviors a patient wants to increase (e.g., going to the park with a son or daughter, taking a walk with the dog or going outside during a lunch break). Measurement also helps the patient assess the level of impact a new behavior exerts on a problem. For example, a patient may find that walking once a week has a positive impact on their well-being, while walking three times a week improves their physical stamina, mood, and sense of well-being.

Feasibility is an important consideration in planning the behavioral experiment. It requires the clinician to balance between pursuing a plan that is sufficiently intense enough to impact on the problem and other factors, including patient motivation and patient resources. The clinician is wise to ask, "What does the plan require and does the patient have the motivation and resources to do it?"

A feasible plan is one that the patient has the skills, resources, and motivation to implement. Of course, a strong plan is relevant to the patient's values, and this has been the subject of extensive discussion in earlier sections of this chapter. Timely plans are those that are important to the patient's life at the present moment in time and in proper amounts of time. For example, a goal that doesn't include a specific start date and a specific number of minutes of engagement in a goal activity (e.g., take a morning walk this week) is less strong than one that does (e.g., take a 10-minute walk at 7:00 AM on Tuesday and Thursday mornings). Consider another example: a patient struggling with the start of recommended physical therapy exercises after a knee surgery. A good plan indicates a starting date and time and other time specifics, such as number of repetitions, (minimum and maximum). SMART is a smart checklist for clinicians to use in progressing toward mastery of skills for planning behavioral experiments that are clearly understood. Let's look at how the clinicians use SMART to develop strong behavioral experiments for Bob and Amy.

Amy's Behavioral Experiment

As readers will recall, the clinician and Amy have explored two possible routines that Amy might use in a behavioral experiment: one to address the sick feeling that led her to leave school without permission and a second to help her sleep more restfully at night.

Clinician: So, what do you think? Two new routines to experiment with: the three breaths and hands-on-heart, kind words routine and then the chill routine before bed. Think they might be helpful?

Amy: Yes, I'll try them.

Clinician: Great. Let's get specific about the details now and make some notes. Do you want to be the note-taker or shall I?

Amy: I will.

Clinician: So, I think that it will help if you practice your breathing and imagination routine before you need to use it, like when you get the sick feeling. Does that make sense?

Amy: Of course, you have to practice anything to get good at it.

Clinician: So, when can you practice it and for how long and how often?

Amy: I like it, so I think I could do it before I go to bed and when I wake up. Why not—it will probable help me.

Clinician: So, will you write that down-AM and PM practice: three breathes, image of your brother's sweet face, and hand on your heart and assurance, "I'm a sweet sister".

Amy: Yes, I can (writing on a sticky note).

Clinician: So how about the night routine? What will that look like?

Amy: The details, huh? Well, I put Sam to bed at 8:30. I'll study until 9:30, but I'll listen to music, classical or boring talk radio on low volume. I won't use my phone or the television since they have that light thing. What else did you say might help?

Clinician: Exercise after school. Maybe something relaxing after your finish studying, like a shower or some stretching.

Amy: Sam likes dancing and wants to learn hip hop so we could do that with some videos and music after school. I'm not sure about the relaxing thing, so maybe I'll just do the other things and see if they help.

Clinician: Perfect. Let's do the what, when, how much details on the second routine, the one after school.

Clinician: (turns to complete chart note while Amy writes) ...

Amy: So here it is, and I got to go. But, just one more thing, can you write a note to the school and say something like I was sick but I'm okay now and shouldn't get expelled or anything-please?

Clinician: Of course, I'll write the note now, give you a copy and email it over to the school. And one more thing concerning our plan, "How confident are you that you will do it? One is no, I won't do it, and ten is yes, I will do it."

Amy: 10, thanks for helping me today.

Clinician: (writing note for school) ... When would you like to check back with the clinic?

Amy: How about I just call if I need to come back.

Clinician: That's fine, Amy. I'd like to see you again and I have same-day appointments available so you can just come when you like. And this is my last question, "How helpful was our visit today? One is not helpful and 10 is very helpful."

Amy: 10! Thanks.

Amy's Behavioral Experiment (written):

AM and PM: three breathes out, Sam, heart, sweet sister
Evening: Dance with Sam Tuesday and Thursday, screens off at 8:30, study until 9:30 or 10

The clinician allowed Amy to be in charge of the specifics of the evolving plan, and this proved helpful to their moving quickly to a plan that was specific, had some measurable components, was within her skill range, was related to her values, and was timely. Amy's commitment to practice the safety routine could make the difference in her ability to work with triggers at school that could jeopardize her future goals. Amy now had a helpful adult in her life that she trusted and could access on a same-day basis. This might be just what she needed to move toward flourishing.

Bob's Behavioral Experiment

Bob and his clinician created a strong values context for designing a behavioral experiment to address his problems with work, family, and health.

Bob: Yeah, that's right. Respect and problem solving are important to me.

Clinician: And that's why the work problem matters so much to you. What does your heart say that you should do at this point?

Bob: Well, be stronger at work and try to help the new manager more. And do more for the people I care about – like the things you have on the list—Sunday games with my son and Tuesday movies with my wife.

Clinician: Awesome, Bob. I'm making some notes here on this sticky. I'll give it to you in minute and I'll write it on the computer too. There's Tuesday movies with your wife, Sunday games with your son. Then, you said you wanted to help your manager more. What would that look like?

Bob: Well, I guess I could offer to help rather than waiting for him to mess up and call me in.

Clinician: Are you meaning you'd just check in with him in the morning when you arrive and let him know you were available to help?

Bob: I could do that and that would be different ... I think I've been sitting at the counter, wondering if the axe would fall today.

Clinician: Understandable. Okay, now I added a quick offer of help to manager in the morning to our list. Take a look, does this look right to you?

Bob: Yep, that's it.

Clinician: So, here's a big question, Bob. How confident are you that you'll do these three things? One is not confident, won't do it and ten is very confident, I'll do it.

Bob: Rating scales ... okay, say eight.

Clinician: Great, Bob. When would you like to check in again?

Bob: Maybe 2 weeks. That'll give me a chance to see how this works.

Clinician: Sounds good; you can book on your way out or call when you want to come in – I have same day appointments. And one last question, "How helpful was your visit today? 1 is not helpful and 10 is very helpful,

Bob: Glad you ask because it was helpful, eight again. Thanks for not bugging me about my weight.

Bob's Behavioral Experiment (written):

> *AM: Quick offer of help to manager*
> *Tuesday's movie with wife*
> *Sunday's game with son*

The clinician developed a SMART behavioral experiment with Bob, and it seemed to better engage Bob in PC. He is probably much more likely to use his team for behavior change support to improve his physical health in future visits.

Metaphors

Metaphors are great intervention strategies as they encourage the patient to take a new perspective on their problems, and they tend to make it easy for clinicians to target all three pillars of psychological flexibility. They also work well in team-based care as all team members can speak to patients using the same metaphor, and this helps decrease the amount of time needed to set up design of behavioral experiments, once the initial metaphor is in place. Patients also appreciate the continuity of care made possible when all members of the HC team use the same language in supporting their new perspective and on-going efforts to improve their health and quality of life. In this section, readers will learn about the *bull's-eye metaphor* and the *life path metaphor*.

Case examples introduced in Chap. 4, provide opportunities for illustrating the use of the bull's-eye and life path metaphors in this chapter. The clinician working with Mary used the bull's-eye in developing a behavior change plan. For Bob, the clinician used the life path metaphor to develop a behavioral experiment in a follow-up visit. Of note, while the bull's-eye and life path are well-known metaphors and used often in FACT work, there are as many other possible metaphors as there are patients and clinicians. Why? Because both clinician and patients can spontaneously co-create metaphors during the course of the clinical conversation. The use of metaphors is one of the most creative aspects of working from a FACT perspective. Clinicians may use any metaphor at any time to help a patient develop a new perspective on their life; a metaphor can create a new context for the problem and promote helpful shifts in perspective.

For example, a clinician might suggest that a patient see their thoughts and feelings as if they were clouds in the spacious blue sky. With the support of this image, the patient may, for a moment, see their struggles from a "sky perspective". The skills involved in allowing thoughts to come and go are important components of connecting and re-connecting with the present moment and cultivating new relationships with difficult thoughts and feelings.

Another example of using a metaphor to enhance a patient's skills in the *Open* and *Aware* pillars is describing a patient's self-critical thoughts and hurt feelings as pieces on a giant checker board, where there are many games and the winners and losers change continuously. Board level is the perspective of a patient's wiser self, the human that can hold all thoughts and feelings and, at the same time, do what matters when it matters. In offering this metaphor, clinicians can begin an on-going conversation with patients about the importance of learning new skills for working well with our busy human minds. Intentional practice of being at board level makes going to board level more accessible when the board level perspective is most needed.

Metaphors are often more powerful than straight-forward psychoeducational explanations about psychological flexibility. They create anchors for new internal behavior and create short-cuts for patients and clinicians to use in communication in future visits (e.g., "How's the sky been? Any interesting weather lately?"). While working towards spontaneous creation of metaphors, clinicians may want to read more about commonly used metaphors in behavior change visits. A good source for this information is the book, *The Big Book of ACT Metaphors: A Practitioner's Guide to Experiential Exercises and Metaphors in Acceptance and Commitment Therapy* (Stoddard & Afari, 2014). Let's take a look at two metaphors that are useful in PC: The Bull's-Eye and the Life Path.

Bull's-Eye

The bull's-eye metaphor guides clinicians toward working with all of the pillars of psychological flexibility. This is helpful to clinicians who are new to using metaphors in the FACT visits. As newbies, there is a tendency to focus on one pillar, and,

Table 5.4 Bull's-eye plan worksheet

1. Begin the conversation by asking what value seems most important to the patient as a guide to working with the problem. Ask the patient to talk more about that value, identifying a time in their life when that value inspired them. When they talk about the memory, slow the pace of the interview and encourage them to attend to thoughts and feelings that show up. Ask for more details. Often, patients will experience emotion and, if so, encourage them to allow it and use it to fuel actions they may want to take at this point in life.
2. Reflect on what you hear and then write a statement on the Bull's-Eye plan using words and images the patient used when talking about the value.
3. Explain that the bull's-eye on the target represents the strongest connection possible between a behavior representing a value and the experience of the value. Explain that the purpose of the bull's-eye is to direct our attention or focus. Most people do not hit the target day in and day out. However, having a target helps us make daily choices with more awareness and attention and "get on the target".
4. Ask the patient to choose a number to represent how close to the bull's-eye value statement their behavior has come, on average, over the past 2 weeks (1 is outer circle and 7 is bull's-eye).
5. Ask the patient to plan a specific behavioral experiment to do in the next 2 weeks; one that they believe would tell them that they are on target and perhaps have moved closer to the bull's-eye than their average for the past 2 weeks.
6. If time allows, ask the patient to anticipate possible barrier(s) to their implementing the plan and teach a skill to help the patient work with an anticipated barrier. Barriers are often related to skill deficits in one or more pillars of psychological flexibility.
7. At follow-up, ask the patient to make a mark on the target to indicate consistency between behaviors and the targeted value. Discuss their experience with the plan. Identify barrier(s) to implementing the plan and teach skills that address the barrier(s). Then, plan another behavioral experiment to help the patient flourish.

often, it is the pillar of Engaged. Many of the interventions that promote *Engagement* are more transparent and therefore approachable. The Bull's-eye metaphor goes with this tendency (i.e., suggesting the start of the intervention with a values discussion) and builds out toward interventions that focus on the *Aware* and *Open* Pillars (i.e., through exploration of barriers to value-consistent action). There are two practice support tools in this chapter for clinicians to use in learning to work with the Bull's-eye metaphor (the Bull's-Eye Plan Worksheet: Table 5.4, and the Bull's-Eye Plan: Fig. 5.1). The Worksheet provides detailed guidance, beginning with starting a conversation that introduces the Bull's-eye to the patient and concluding with how to using the Bull's-eye in follow-up visits. Once established, the Bull's-eye becomes a tool for the clinician and patient to use over time to support behavior change.

Most patients readily understand what a target and bull's-eye are, so patients are easily engaged in a conversation about it. The very act of introducing the bull's-eye encourages patients to shift toward a less literal and more contemplative perspective on their lives. Teammates learn the bull's-eye readily, given its transparency, and this allows for continuity of care, as all team members may inquire about the Bull's-eye and related plans. One team member may follow-up the work of another team member by evaluating the impact of a plan from a previous visit, teaching skills that help address barriers to behavior change and developing new behavioral experiments.

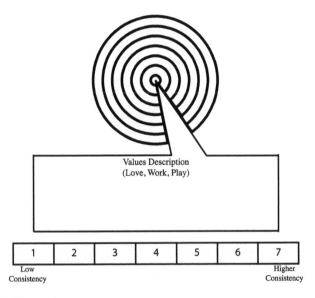

Fig. 5.1 The bull's-eye plan

While the bull's-eye may be a useful metaphor with almost any patient, it is particularly useful for patients attempting to make and sustain multiple behavior changes, such as patients challenged with self-managing chronic conditions. The bull's-eye may be used as a care plan and even integrated into the *Electronic Health Record* (EHR) to encourage a common language between the patient and team members, one that focuses on value and small changes over time. The case of Mary provides an opportunity to demonstrate the use of the Bull's-Eye Plan as a care plan.

As illustrated in the following dialogue, the clinician used the bull's-eye to encourage Mary's connection with her values, so that they were powerful enough to fuel a more vital course of action at an important choice point in life. As the reader may recall from the contextual interview with Mary in Chap. 4, she agreed that "caring" was an important value for her and said that she wanted to choose "Caring, calling, and hurting" instead of "stuck, watching tele, and not feeling". The clinician used the bull's eye plan to develop a behavioral experiment with Mary (Fig. 5.2, Mary's Bull's-Eye Plan).

Clinician: So, Mary, this is a target and the center of a target is called … what?
Mary: The bull's-eye.
Clinician: Right. We are going to use this bull's-eye idea to get you moving … moving in the direction of what and who matters. In this case, the value that seems to be calling for your attention is caring, and the person inspiring you is Lucy. So caring is an action and we'll need to figure out what actions you want to engage in to show that you care.
Mary: Right. I call Lucy because I care about her and I go to work because I care about the people there.

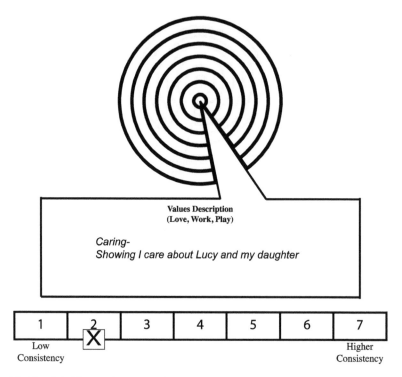

Fig. 5.2 Mary's bull's-eye plan (Example)

Clinician: Yes, you already do things that show you care, and I think you heart is
   telling you that you have more caring to do. The question is what one or two
   things in the way of your daily or weekly activities might you do now to
   strengthen your experience of caring? And by the way, Mary, I want you to know
   that there is nothing too small to consider. In fact, small changes are powerful
   because that's what gets us started moving on the path we want to take.

Mary: Well, it would be easy for me to start writing Lucy and my daughter, too, a
   letter every week.

Clinician: Great. I bet they would like that. Anything else come to mind?

Mary: Well, I said I would go through William's clothes and donate things I thought
   other people could use. I know that he would like that; he was a generous person,
   always able to think about other people. I just don't know if I can do that …
   (looking down, beginning to cry …)

Clinician: Would that be more do-able if you did it with your daughter?

Mary: Yes, I think so. I guess maybe the first step would be to ask my daughter to
   help me with it.

Clinician: I like it – we are talking about two experiments that you think would
   bring you closer to your bull's-eye of caring: writing the letters and talking with
   your daughter about sorting out William's belongings. If you did those things, do
   you think they would move you a little closer to your bull's-eye?

Mary: Yes, I think so.

Clinician: Great. Just a couple of more questions. First, I want to ask you to indicate the extent to which your day-to-day actions have been consistent with your values over the past 2 weeks. Just make a mark on the target (handing Mary a pen). This is our baseline, where we are starting with our first dart, so to speak. When you return, you will make another mark and we'll see if our plan is moving you toward your bull's eye.

Mary: That makes sense. If I want to get on target, and I have to get started.

Clinician: Mary, nobody is living their values all the time, that's why we need a target. Even when we have a target to direct our efforts, our aim varies. Somedays, we are closer to the bull's-eye and some days we are further way. Big losses in life set most us back for a while. And, Mary, you already do things that get you on target on Sundays, right?

Mary: Oh, yes, when I call Lucy, I'm on target. And I am going to write that precious little girl a letter as soon as I get home. The thought of it warms my heart.

Clinician: Warms mine, too, Mary. I'm going to have Alice, our team nurse, give you a call in a week to see how your bull's-eye work is going, and then I'd like to see you back in a couple of weeks. One last thing … I'm wondering if you would be willing to try sleeping in your bed for a few nights, maybe just listening to relaxing music and resting in your bed for a few nights. You know, an experiment, to see if you feel a little more rested the next day. More rest means more energy for caring (winking).

Mary: Yes, I'll do that. I had been thinking about it but I don't know I just hadn't done it yet.

Clinician: So, what will your letter writing day be?

Mary: Today – well, let's just make it Fridays, since I feel like writing today.

Clinician: And what two nights will you experiment with resting in your bed, say starting around 10 PM?

Mary: I'll try it tonight and Saturday night and maybe I won't feel so tired when I call Lucy on Sunday. Clinician: So, here's what I've written on our sticky note. Does this say it right?

Mary's behavioral experiment (written):

Friday: Letter writing, Mary and daughter
Friday and Saturday: Resting in bed for a while, starting at 10 PM
Sunday: Call Lucy

Mary: Yes, that's right. Do I keep this?

Clinician: Yes, you do. And, Mary, tell me how confident you are that you'll do these things? One means no, you won't do them and 10 means yes, you are very confident that you will do them.

Mary: 10, I will doctor.

Clinician: And last question, how helpful was our visit today? One means not helpful and ten means very helpful.

Mary: That's 10, too. Thank you.

The clinician used the bull's-eye skillfully to help Mary recover from grief and move toward flourishing. The clinician also planned timelier follow-up, using a team member to check-on the bull's-eye plan. This is an important aspect of care for more vulnerable patients.

Life Path

The life path metaphor (Fig. 5.3) is a powerful option for patients needing to make a choice and turn in a new direction. It offers them the choice of using more of their energy to approach and pursue what matters and less in controlling difficult thoughts and feelings. When using metaphor, clinicians often start with a focus on the *Aware* pillar, a good place to start when patients are distressed and lost in thought about the past and worries about the future. Awareness is of fundamental importance to a patient in need of a new perspective on difficult feelings and thoughts that are pushing them around and consuming too much of their energy. With a more workable distance for viewing their psychological pain, patients are more able to develop a sense of acceptance and even compassion for themselves as they come to perceive the connection between their pain and what matters to them. Awareness is also of pivotal importance in further clarifying values and in making moment-to-moment choices to engage in new approach-oriented behaviors.

This chapter offers two practice support tools for readers to use in learning to work with the life path metaphor. The *Life Path Plan Worksheet* (Table 5.5) provides a list of questions the clinician may pose to the patient during the course of a life path intervention. The list is inspirational, and clinicians may find other ways of wording the questions in order to connect more strongly with a patient. This worksheet may also be used by patients participating in a life path class. More information about using this metaphor in a class in available (see Strosahl, Robinson & Gustavsson, 2012) and materials are available on this books website (see basicsofbehaviorchangeinprimarycare.com).

The second practice support tool is the *Life Path Plan* (Fig. 5.3), which can be used to guide an intervention where the clinician and patient work together using the guide as a focus for their conversation. Alternatively, the clinician may take the metaphor to a new level by physicalizing it. In this deployment, the clinician would ask the patient to stand and imagine a path, perhaps between one wall and the opposing wall. One side would represent what and who matters and the other, the patient's control efforts. This promotes greater awareness and a deeper emotional experience, as the patient turns and looks one way and the other, describing and deciding.

The following segment of clinician-patient interaction illustrates use of the life path metaphor in a follow-up (Fig. 5.3, Bob's life path Plan). Bob returned with his wife; he reported improvement in his work situation and in his family relationships. He and his wife wanted to talk about ways to help him improve his health. Now that he was feeling better, he was more concerned about his blood pressure, which had always been difficult to control. He wanted to live a long life, and he and his wife had been talking about the things they wanted to do together in retirement.

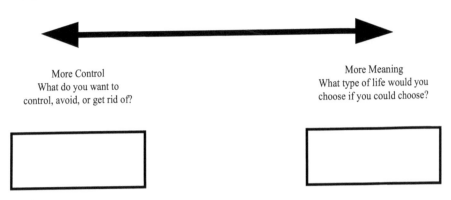

More Control
What do you want to
control, avoid, or get rid of?

More Meaning
What type of life would you
choose if you could choose?

1. Where are you on your life path? Mark an X. Which direction are you moving toward?

2. What, if any, are the costs and benefits of moving towards control?

3. Why would you want to move toward your values now? What values?

4. What behaviors would tell you that you're moving toward more meaning in life?

5. How would you turn in the direction of a more meaningful life?

6. When you turn toward control, how will you know to turn toward meaning?

7. Who or what helps you move in the direction of more meaning?

Fig. 5.3 The life path plan. (Adapted from Strosahl, Robinson & Gustavsson, 2012 Choosing: My Life Path and Turn-Around)

Clinician: Hey, Bob, good to see you and glad to see you brought your wife, today.

Bob: Yes, my better half, Liz.

Clinician: Hi, Liz, welcome. Bob, I want to check in on the work stress. On our scale of one to ten where one is not a problem and ten is a very big problem, how big of a problem is work stress now.

Bob: Better. I'm getting a relationship with the new guy. He's using me a lot more and has even given me some new responsibilities that I like.

Clinician: Got a number?

Bob: Oh, sure, say 4. I guess I still wonder what will happen and of course I miss my old friend, the previous owner.

Table 5.5 The life path plan worksheet

1. How long have you had the problem that brings you here?
With this question, the clinician is inviting the patient to look at the problem from a different perspective, a view that encourages them to step back and look at their life over a longer period of time. The clinician might use the metaphor of an "eagles eye view versus a mouse view".
2. What have you tried? Helpful results? Less helpful results?
The clinician is attempting to identify the patient's efforts to solve the problem and how these efforts have impacted the problem and the patient's ability to flourish. Many times, patients have found ways to control or diminish difficult thoughts and feelings on a short-term basis. These strategies may have costs or unanticipated negative consequences. If so, what?
3. What do you want from life?
Here, the clinician is attempting to engage the patient in a conversation about the values that are most important at this moment in their life.
4. What are the barriers to doing what you want in life?
The clinician is attempting to help the patient identify reasons, rules and stories that play a role in maintaining the status quo. Patients may be able to hear themselves in a new way, as they recount reasons thry've never questioned or tell stories that they may be able to experience now with a different perspective. The clinician might suggest that barriers may include things the patient is doing to avoid or control difficult feelings and thoughts.
5. What do you do when the barriers show up?
What most patients do when barriers show up is to control them (e.g., "try not to think about it" or "do something to distract myself").
6. Are you at war with the barriers? What are the consequences of being "at war" with the barriers?
When a patient is at war, they are probably using most of their resources for control and avoidance. They may be unable to connect with their values and see the possibility of more approach-oriented behavior. If this is the case, the clinician will try to help the patient find a way to "turn-around", even a little, so that a connection with values is possible, and to let the barriers come with them as they turn. The clinician will help the client have the barriers in a way that requires less effort and less struggle. The patient can learn to notice and name barriers rather than fight them, freeing energy for pursuing what matters.

Clinician: Of course. So how did it go with the plan: Family activities on Sunday and Tuesday and the morning check-in with the manager. All good?

Bob: Yes, no problem. Did them all and they helped, but today Liz and I want to talk about how to get my health better. We've been talking about 5 years from now and retiring. We both love to travel and we want to go to some of the national parks. Hike around and see the sites.

Clinician: That sounds great.

Bob: Yes, and I found my blood pressure cuff and I've been checking it and it's pretty high at times. That scares me and Liz and so I want to get a plan to do better with food and exercise. We want to do it together, right Liz?

Liz: Yes, that's right. I've been nagging Bob for years and that doesn't work. I could stand to improve my health habits, too. We get the American Association of Retired Persons newsletter, and they have lots of good ideas and say it's never too late (smiling).

Clinician: Okay, I have an idea. Let's do an exercise together. Stand up, the two of you and stand here in the middle of the room. On this wall, let's imagine there's a window that opens to the vision of you two at a national park ... you're hiking around together, seeing the beauty of nature and enjoying your partnership. Now on this other wall (pointing to the opposite wall), there is a box on the floor full of things that you don't want. Not sure about what's in that bucket, but maybe thoughts like, "I shouldn't have to deprive myself of desserts. I must have seconds on that pasta. I'm too tired to go for a walk today." Any of those sound familiar?

Liz: I think you are reading our minds.

Clinician: And maybe there's feelings, like sadness and irritability, and things you do to get away from all that thinking and feeling, like turning on the television.

Bob: Oh, yes, that sounds like our lives and our home. Right, Liz? So, what's next, doc?

Clinician: Well, I think it's about learning how to have those thoughts and feelings and still do things daily that prepare you for your healthy future. Like to just be able to notice them and not let them control you. If you could just notice them and give them a name—the "don't wants" or something like that. Then, you could just say, hey let's take our "don't wants" and go for our after-dinner walk. Something like that.

Bob: Hmm. Never thought of that. What do you think, Liz? Take the "don't wants" and just do it (winks at Liz).

Liz: I like it.

Clinician: Okay, we are getting to the point where I can start writing out a plan. What shall I put on it? What sort of things would you be doing if you turned toward "seeing the national parks together"? What steps do you want to take together now on your life path.

Bob: (looking at Liz) ... the walking after dinner is a good idea. Liz likes that – she often takes about a 15-minute walk. And I think it would be easiest for me if we just took sugar out of the house. If it's there, I'll eat it.

Liz: I agree Bob; I can clean it out today. It'll be better for us.

Clinician: Those are great starts. Maybe we will stop there for now ... just see how those go for a week and then add something new. It's funny how doing one health-promoting thing tends to lead to doing another. Bob, I'm writing a second blood pressure medicine for you ... I'd like you to try it and continue to take your blood pressure once in the morning and once at night. I'll ask Judy, my nurse, to call you in a week to see how the numbers are looking. Hey, you two – keep your eyes open for the "don't wants".

In a short visit, the clinician used the life path metaphor to help Bob and Liz plan a few new steps on their life path and use a new skill in working with difficult thoughts and feelings they had been at war with for years. There are many angles to explore when using the life path metaphor. There are video demonstrations of the life path intervention, as well as the bull's eye intervention, available on the basicsofbehaviorchangeinprimarycare.com and create hyperlink to all references to the website in the book (basicsofbehaviorchangeinprimarycare.com) for readers that want to learn more. Metaphors, like the life path and bull's-eye, are great options for promoting powerful behavior change in PC.

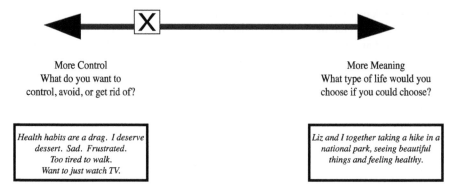

More Control	More Meaning
What do you want to control, avoid, or get rid of?	What type of life would you choose if you could choose?

Health habits are a drag. I deserve dessert. Sad. Frustrated. Too tired to walk. Want to just watch TV.

Liz and I together taking a hike in a national park, seeing beautiful things and feeling healthy.

1. Where are you on your life path? Mark an X. Which direction are you moving toward?

   Facing more meaning; motivated

2. What, if any, are the costs and benefits of moving towards control?

   Getting worse, gain more weight, feeling more tierd, blood presue and all that worse

3. Why would you want to move toward your values now? What values?

   Liz and I want to do this together, for our health now and for our future

4. What behaviors would tell you that you're moving toward more meaning in life?

   Getting the sugar out of the house; walking after dinner

5. How would you turn in the direction of a more meaningful life?

   Just say we can take the "don't wants" with us and "just do it"

6. When you turn toward control, how will you know to turn toward meaning?

   Forget that the "don't wants" are "just don't wants" and start believing them again, letting them push us around

7. Who or what helps you move in the direction of more meaning?

   Liz, my son too

Fig. 5.4 Bob's life path plan (Example). (Adapted from Strosahl, Robinson & Gustavsson, 2012 (Choosing: My Life Path and Turn-Around))

Working Smart in Primary Care

In this short section, readers learn about strategies to pursue to further the reach of their efforts to help people make meaningful change to their behavior. Historically, the penetration of contextual behavioral science into the worldwide population has been minimal and by working in the context of PC, you precious reader, can change that. In addition to using powerful assessment and intervention strategies, you will need to explore other tactics, and this section suggest three important directions. Using assistants to help with clinical work and thinking beyond clinic visits and the one-to-one contact are ways to enhance patient access to behavior change services.

Use Assistants

Not all behavioral change interventions require delivery by a licensed healthcare provider. Behavioral health clinician assistants, medical assistants, community health workers, promotores, and others can assist with this work. They can shorten the amount of time required by licensed healthcare workers by completing pre-visit surveys and by teaching interventions, particularly in languages that they can speak but the licensed healthcare provider does not. They can improve efficiency by managing same-day visits and assisting with charting. They also can provide critical support in delivery of group-based services, particularly group medical visits which may serve up to 20 patients. Assistants may also provide important timely phone support, particularly for more vulnerable patients.

Think Beyond Clinic Visits

The world of the Internet grows daily, expanding the methods for delivery of behavior change services exponentially. Clinicians working in PC can connect patients with evidence-based Internet services and encourage them to complete on-line behavior change programs. Increasingly, clinicians will be able to connect with patients in need of behavior change through video services, computer portals, and telehealth cabins. Readers need to explore and expand options for vitual healthcare visits that encourage health behavior change.

Think Beyond the One-to-One

Since many, many patients need support in making and maintaining behavior changes, clinicians need to prepare to deliver services in group formats. Group services may include workshops with a prevention focus (e.g., a workshop for tweens and parents focused on preparing for the solicitations of companies selling electronic tobacco products), acute services (e.g., for the many people struggling with the loss of loved ones to the opioid epidemic), and chronic care services (e.g., group medical visits for the almost one in ten Americans with diabetes). Low intensity group interventions using *Acceptance and Commitment Therapy* (ACT) (Hayes, Strosahl, & Wilson, 2012) are well received by patients struggling with medical and psychological problems and associated with improved clinical outcomes (Dindo,

2015). Group services also offer members of the PC team with different training backgrounds the chance to work together, to learn from each other, and to find and refine a common voice that prioritizes and promotes behavior change.

Making Progress Over Time

This book introduced many Contextual Behavioral Science (CBS) strategies for promoting behavior change in PC. Appendix A provides a checklist for readers to use to assess learning, plan a course of study, and monitor progress. Review the "Contextual Behavioral Scientist Check-In" on a regular basis, and remember, "Where attention goes, energy flows".

Strategies for Delivering Powerful Behavior Change Interventions

There are nine strategies for readers to review in Table 5.6, A Checklist of Recommended Strategies for Providing Powerful Behavior Change Interventions. They are explained in the following section. Select a few initial targets to pursue, ones that seem important and feasible for your work at this time. Later, select additional strategies, so that you continue to build your skills for helping patients make powerful changes in their behavior.

1. *Help a patient make gains in psychological flexibility during a visit.* Developing a simple, straight-forward behavioral experiment in a 10-minute visit can boost a patient's psychological flexibility. Goal setting is pretty clear cut, and singles, as you will recall, are great when time is limited. When you have a little more time, think about the pillars and try to influence patient psychological flexibility during the visit. Remember the FACT *Pillars Intervention Guide* in Table 5.1 and refer back to it often.
2. *Let patients know that failure is a great way to learn.* Remember that some patients fear failure more than others. Explain the usefulness of failure when one fails mindfully.
3. *Develop written behavior change experiments in all visits and assure patient confidence in implementing the experiment.* If the patient voices a confidence rating of less than seven, revise the plan. Write the plan (or have the patient write it) on a small piece of paper so that the patient is more likely to keep it with them (for example, in a wallet). Changing the plan to get a higher confidence rating requires less than 2 minutes most of the time; so, do it.
4. *Use CBT interventions (such as Cognitive Behavioral Therapy-Insomnia, problem solving therapy, behavioral activation, progressive muscle relaxation and behavioral parent training).* They are evidence-based, brief, and well-received by patients! Read more about CBT; it is a close relative of FACT and offers many evidence-based processes. This books website offers a variety of CBT patient

education materials, as well as coaching on the use of these materials (see basicsofbehaviorchangeinprimarycare.com)

5. *Use metaphors, like the life path.* It targets all three pillars of psychological flexibility and promotes radical behavior change. Some clinicians will love metaphors and find it easy to think of them spontaneously in-patient visits; others may want to read more about these powerful approaches to behavior change.

6. *Use metaphors, like the bull's-eye.* They are useful in team-based care for patients with chronic conditions. Hopefully, readers will look for a teammate that's interested in starting group medical visits for patients with chronic pain or diabetes. The bull's-eye metaphor is an excellent anchor for behavior change in on-going monthly group care services.

7. *Use group behavior change interventions to increase the penetration of behavioral health services to the clinic population, decrease costs, and improve efficiency.* Remember that groups can be one and done (e.g., a three-hour workshop focused on the life path metaphor for parents of children on the autism spectrum, a two-hour workshop on family meal time). Alternatively, group services may consist of a series of classes, where patients learn skills. Be sure to market group services as classes and allow same-day access.

8. *Use assistants to extend your ability to provide behavioral healthcare to more patients.* Assistants may help with clinic, phone and home visits. They can learn behavior change protocols and deliver interventions with supervision and consultation from a licensed healthcare clinician.

9. *Use the Contextual Behavioral Scientist Check-In (CBSC) to monitor your progress in learning to promote powerful behavior change interventions.* Chapters 3, 4, and 5, introduced readers to the tools of *Contextual Behavioral Science* (CBS).

Table 5.6 Checklist: Recommended strategies for providing powerful behavior change interventions[a]

Selected strategy	Recommended strategies
	1. Help a patient make gains in psychological flexibility during a visit.
	2. Let patients know that failure is a great way to learn.
	3. Develop written behavior change experiments in all visit and assure patient confidence in implementing the experiment.
	4. Use CBT interventions (such as Cognitive Behavioral Therapy-insomnia, problem solving therapy, behavioral activation, progressive muscle relaxation and behavioral parent training).
	5. Use metaphors, like the life path.
	6. Use metaphors, like the bull's-eye.
	7. Use group behavior change interventions to increase the penetration of behavioral health services to the clinic population, decrease costs, and improve efficiency.
	8. Use assistants to extend your ability to provide behavioral healthcare to more patients.
	9. Use the CBSC to monitor your progress in learning to promote powerful behavior change interventions.

[a]Place a mark beside strategies that you believe would be helpful in your clinic and feasible at this point in time.

The CBS approach grows from behavioral psychology and adds in new ways of looking at the human situation. It focuses on understanding what is important to patients and how what they do works to support or not support what is important to them. With CBS tools, readers are empowered to help patients pursue the lives they want and deserve with precision, scope and depth. Use the *CBSC* in Appendix A to self-assess your skills and plan targets for growth over time. It's a good idea to set a reminder in your calendar to complete it again 3 months from now.

Summary

The goal of this chapter was to empower clinicians to work together in developing strong behavior change interventions with patients and supporting them overtime. Behavioral interventions include those that focus on skill training in clinic visits and those that focus on developing behavioral experiments that target behavioral variability in the patient's home, work or school setting, and community. Patients are most likely to implement behavioral experiments that are feasible and related to their values; no behavior change is too small if it relates to the patient's values and is pursued with confidence.

Review

1. Psychological flexibility can be enhanced in brief contextual visits.
2. Behavioral experiments need to be engaging and SMART.
3. Metaphors, like the Life Path and bull's-eye, encourage the clinician to work on all three pillars of psychological flexibility.
4. In order to increase the reach of behavioral science, clinicians need to explore use of assistants, group-based services, and all of the newly emerging venues made possible by new technologies.

Table 5.7 Tips for leaders

1. Explore building interventions, like the bull's-eye, into the *Electronic Health Record* (EHR) to function as care plans.
2. Support use of registries of patients receiving behavioral health services in the contexts of group medical visits, such as those with chronic or persistent pain.
3. Create reports that provide feedback to clinicians on visit length and change in BH measure scores from the initial to the follow-up visit.
4. Create reports that detail the impact of delivery of BH services on key primary care metrics, such as percentage of patients with acceptable levels of diabetic control or change in Body Mass Index (BMI).
5. Encourage teams to develop programs that achieve the quadruple aim, like group medical visits that provide both behavior change support and medical services.

5. Skills for developing powerful behavior change interventions develop over time with continued study and practice. Table 5.5 provides a Checklist of Recommended Strategies for Providing Powerful Behavior Change Interventions. Readers can use it to choose several strategies for further study and intentional practice over time.
6. Clinicians need leadership support, and Table 5.7 (Tips for Leaders) provides suggestions for the clinic leadership group. Informed leaders are more able to support behavioral intervention services.

References

Cigrang, J. A., Rauch, S. A., Avila, L. L., Bryan, C. J., Goodie, J. L., Hryshko-Mullen, A., & Peterson, A. L.. & STRONG STAR Consortium (2011). Treatment of active-duty military with PTSD in primary care: Early findings. *Psychological Services, 8*(2), 104–113.

Dindo, L. (2015). One-day acceptance and commitment training workshops in medical populations. *Current Opinions in Psychology, 2*, 38–42. https://doi.org/10.1016/jcopsye.2015.018.

Dobmeyer, A. E. (2018). *Psychological treatments of medical patients in integrated primary care. Clinical health psychology series.* Washington, DC: American Psychological Association.

Gallimore, C., Corso, K. A., Robinson, P. J., & Runyan, C. N. (2018). Pharmacists in primary care: Lessons learned from integrated behavioral health. *Medical Practice Management*, 321–325.

Glover, N. G., Sylvers, P. D., Shearer, E. M., Kane, M.-C., Clasen, P. C., Epler, A. J., … Bonow, J. T. (2016). The efficacy of focused acceptance and commitment therapy in VA primary care. *Psychological Services, 13*(2), 156–161.

Goodie, J., Isler, W., Hunter, C., & Peterson, A. (2009). Using behavioral health consultants to treat insomnia in primary care: A clinical case series. *Journal of Clinical Psychology, 65*, 294–304.

Hayes, S. C., Strosahl, K. D., & Wilson, K. G. (2012). Acceptance and commitment therapy. In *The process and practice of mindful change* (2nd ed.). New york, NY: Guilford.

Hunter, C. L., Funderburk, J. S., Polaha, J., Bauman, D., Goodie, J. L., & Hunter, C. M. (2017a). Primary Care Behavioral Health (PCBH) model research: Current state of the science and a call to action. *Journal of Clinical Psychology in Medical Settings*. Published on-line 03-Oct-2017. https://doi.org/10.1007/s10880-017-9512-0.

Hunter, C. L., Goodie, J. L., Oordt, M. S., & Dobmeyer, A. C. (2017b). *Integrated behavioral health in primary care: Step-by-step guidance for assessment and intervention* (2nd ed.). Washington, DC: American Psychological Association.

Reiter, J. T., Dobmeyer, A. C., & Hunter, C. L. (2017). The primary care behavioral health (PCBH) model: An overview and operational definition. *Journal of Clinical Psychology in Medical Settings, 24*(4). National Committee for Quality Assurance 2011.

Robinson, P., Gould, D., & Strosahl, K. (2010). *Real behavior change in primary care: Improving outcomes and increasing job satisfaction.* Oakland, CA: New Harbinger.

Robinson, P., Von Korff, M., Bush, T., Lin, E. H. B., & Ludman, E. J. (2020). The impact of Primary Care Behavioral Health Services on patient behaviors: A randomized controlled trial. *Family Systems and Health, 38*(1), 6–15. https://www.yourcoach.be/en/coaching-tools/smart-goal-setting.php.

Robinson, P. J., & Reiter, J. T. (2007). *Behavioral consultation and primary care: A guide to integrating services.* New York, NY: Springer Science and Media.

Robinson, P. J., & Reiter, J. T. (2015). *Behavioral consultation and primary care: A guide to integrating services* (2nd ed.). New York, NY: Springer Science and Media.

Starfield, B., Shi, L., & Macinko. (2005). Contribution of primary care to health systems and health. *The Millbank Quarterly: A Multidisciplinary Journal of Population Health and Health Policy, 83*(3), 457–502.

Stoddard, J. A., & Afari, N. (2014). *The big book of metaphors: A practitioner's guide to experiential exercises and metaphors in acceptance and commitment therapy.* Oakland, CA: New Harbinger.

Strosahl, K., Robinson, P., & Gustavsson, T. (2012). *Brief interventions for radical change: Focused acceptance and commitment therapy.* Oakland, CA: New Harbinger.

Strosahl, K. D., & Robinson, P. J. (2018). Adapting empirically supported treatments in the era of integrated care: A roadmap for success. *Clinical Psychology: Science and Practice.* https://doi.org/10.1111/cpsp.12246

Appendix A

Table A.1.1 Contextual behavioral scientist check-in

Use this tool as a check on your fidelity to the approach recommended in this book, *Basics of Behavior Change*. Rate your skill level on a scale where 1 = low skill and 10 = high skill. With more study and practice, you will see your numbers increase!

Skill level today	Skills
	1. Complete a functional assessment.
	2. Complete assessment and intervention in 15–25 min.
	3. Identify patient strengths and use them in interventions and plans.
	4. Understand the difference between behaviors that are actions and behaviors that are thoughts, feelings, and sensations.
	5. Understand the difference between behaviors that support avoidance and behaviors that support approach toward who and what matters.
	6. Have a meaningful conversation with a patient about who and what matters in their life.
	7. Help a patient intentionally respond in a new way to difficult thoughts, feelings, and sensations.
	8. Assist a patient with learning how to contact the present moment and return there intentionally.
	9. Provide behavior change assistance to individuals, couples and families.
	10. Take a team approach to using behavior change to support health and flourishing for all.

Appendix B (Chapter 3 Measures, Tools, Worksheets)

Table B.3.1 The flourishing project measure[a]

Domain	Questions	Score
Happiness and life satisfaction	1. Overall, how satisfied are you with your life as a whole these days? 0 = Not Satisfied at All, 10 = Completely Satisfied 2. In general, how happy or unhappy do you usually feel? 0 = Extremely Unhappy, 10 = Extremely Happy	
Mental and physical health	3. In general, how would you rate your physical health? 0 = Poor, 10 = Excellent 4. How would you rate your overall mental health? 0 = Poor, 10 = Excellent	
Meaning and purpose	5. Overall, to what extent do you feel the things you do in your life are worthwhile? 0 = Not at All Worthwhile, 10 = Completely Worthwhile 6. I understand my purpose in life. 0 = Strongly Disagree, 10 = Strongly Agree	
Character and virtue	7. I always act to promote good in all circumstances, even in difficult and challenging situations. 0 = Not True, 10 = Completely True of Me 8. I am always able to give up some happiness now for greater happiness later. 0 = Not True of Me, 10 = Completely True of Me	
Close social relationships	9. I am content with my friendships and relationships. 0 = Strongly Disagree, 10 = Strongly Agree 10. My relationships are as satisfying as I would want them to be. 0 = Strongly Disagree, 10 = Strongly Agree	
Financial and material stability	11. How often do you worry about being able to meet normal monthly living expenses? 0 = Worry All of the Time, 10 = Do Not Ever Worry 12. How often do you worry about safety, food, or housing? 0 = Worry All of the Time, 10 = Do Not Ever Worry	

[a]Van derWeele, T.J. (2017). On the promotion of human flourishing. Proceedings of the National Academy of Sciences, U.S.A., 31: 8148–8156.

© The Author(s), under exclusive license to Springer Nature Switzerland AG Pte Ltd 2019
P. J. Robinson, *Basics of Behavior Change in Primary Care*, SpringerBriefs in Psychology, https://doi.org/10.1007/978-3-030-32050-8

Table B.3.2 The Acceptance and Action Questionnaire-II (AAQ-II)[a]

Below you will find a list of statements. Please rate how true each statement is for you by using the scale below to fill in your choice

1	2	3	4	5	6	7
Never true	Very seldom true	Seldom true	Sometimes true	Frequently true	Almost always true	Always true
1. My painful experiences and memories make it difficult for me to live a life that I would value.						
2. I'm afraid of my feelings.						
3. I worry about not being able to control my worries and feelings.						
4. My painful memories prevent me from having a fulfilling life.						
5. Emotions cause problems in my life.						
6. It seems like most people are handling their lives better than I am.						
7. Worries get in the way of my success.						
Total Score						

[a]Bond, Hayes, Baer, Carpenter, Guenole, et al. 2011.

Table B.3.3   The approach-avoidance tool

	Avoid	Approach
Actions	What behaviors does the patient do to get away from difficult thoughts, feelings, sensations, and situations (e.g., distracting behaviors, drugs / alcohol, etc.)?	What behaviors does the patient do that are consistent with what matters and who matters?
Thoughts **Feelings** **Sensations**	What thoughts, feelings, and sensations does the patient use to control, ignore, suppress, or avoid? What unworkable rule(s) is the patient following?	What matters to the patient? Who matters to the patient? What helpful rule(s) is the patient following?

Appendix C (Chapter 4 Measures, Tools, Worksheets)

Table C.4.1 Contextual interview questions[a]

Life context: Love, work, play and health	
Love	Where do you live? With whom? How long have you been there? Are things okay at your home? Do you have loving relationships with your family or friends?
Work	Do you work? Study? If yes, what is your work? Do you enjoy it? If not working, are you looking for work? If not working and not looking for a job, how do your support yourself?
Play	What do you do for fun? For relaxation? For connecting with people in your neighborhood or community?
Health	Do you use tobacco products, alcohol, illegal drugs, social media? Do you exercise on a regular basis for your health? Do you eat well? Sleep well?
Problem context: The Three T's	
Time	When did this start? How often does it happen? What happens before / after the problem? Why do you think it is a problem now?
Trigger	Is there anything—a situation or a person—that seems to set it off?
Trajectory	What's this problem been like over time? Have there been times when it was less of a concern? More of a concern? And recently…getting worse, better?
Workability Question	What have you tried (to address the problem)? How has that worked in the short run? In the long run or in the sense of being consistent with what really matters to you?

[a]Adapted from Robinson, Gould, & Strosahl, 2010.

Table C.4.2   Four-square tool[a]

	Avoidance / Controls suffering	Approach / Supports flourishing
Actions		
Thoughts **Emotions** **Sensations**		

[a]Adapted from Strosahl, Robinson, and Gustavsson, 2012.

Table C.4.3 FACT Pillars Assessment Tool (PAT)

Use this tool to assess patient functioning in each pillar and to plan interventions that might promote greater psychological flexibility.

1. What are the patient's strengths and weaknesses?
2. Is there a pillar that is a priority target for skill development at this point in time?

Open	Aware	Engaged
• Accepts distressing thoughts and feelings • Creates a safe observational distance from distressing thoughts and feelings • Uses experiences to inform behavior, rather than habits and rules	• Intentionally focuses on present moment experience • Uses self-reflective awareness to promote sensitivity to context • Can change perspectives on stories told about self and others	• Speaks about values with emotion, recalls moments of values-in-action, and accepts vulnerability that comes with caring • Plans and implements behavior change experiments that promote vitality
Strengths	**Strengths**	**Strengths**
Deficits	**Deficits**	**Deficits**
Targets	**Targets**	**Targets**

Table C.4.4 Rating scale questions[a]

1. How big of a problem is x? 1 = not a problem and 10 = a very big problem
2. How confident are you that you will *do* this experiment? 1 = not confident and 10 = very confident
3. How helpful was this visit? 1 = not helpful and 10 = very helpful

Table C.4.5 Contextual assessment checklist

Do I know:
1. What the patient is doing to address the problem
2. How their solutions are working
3. What matters and who matters to the patient
4. What the patient would do in a world where anything was possible

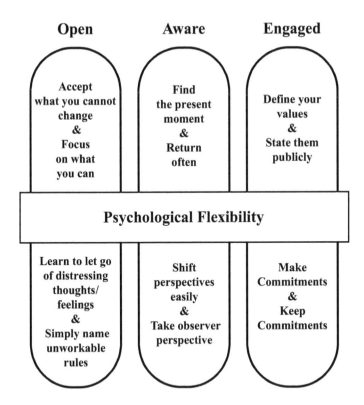

Fig. C.4.1 FACT pillars of flexibility

Appendix D (Chapter 5 Measures, Tools, Worksheets)

Table D.5.1 FACT Pillar Intervention Guide (PIG)

When intervening with patients, use the suggested guides to assist with moment-to-moment interactions that move the patient toward greater psychological flexibility

Open	Aware	Engaged
When "stuck", be curious, model acceptance, notice the "mind"	If confused, go to the present, look at different perspectives	Whenever possible, promote connection between values and action
Support openness and curiosity about previously avoided thoughts/ feelings/ sensations	Promote flexible, voluntary and purposeful attention to the present moment	Identify qualities of meaningful action in the here and now
Attend to thinking as an ongoing process, rather than the world structured by it	Support mindfulness and noticing of the continuity of consciousness	Collaboratively create SMART behavioral experiments

P. J. Robinson, *Basics of Behavior Change in Primary Care*, SpringerBriefs
in Psychology, https://doi.org/10.1007/978-3-030-32050-8

Table D.5.2   The "Relate the Problem to Values" worksheet

Experiment with using one or more of these questions to assist the patient with seeing a
relationship between the problem and values that are important to the patient at this time.

1. Tell me more about why it is important for you to find a new way to address this problem
    now.

2. In a world where anything is possible, what would you do about this problem?

3. If you could make this problem go away, but it cost you the ability to care about problems
    like this, would you?

4. If you didn't have x as value, would this problem matter to you?

5. What does your heart say about this problem?

6. What happens in your body now when we are talking about this?

Consider patient answers to questions asked and conceptualize a plan that would be important to
the patient.

Are there skills that you could teach the patient during the visit to strengthen the patient's
ability to implement the plan?

Table D.5.3   The "SMART Behavioral Experiment" worksheet

Use this worksheet to improve your skills for developing behavioral experiments with patients. If the patient's history included painful punishing experiences (e.g., critical or depressed parent, multiple traumas), you may want to spend a little more time explaining the value of experimenting and the usefulness of trying something new.

A SMART behavioral experiment is engaging and SMART
A. Is the experiment engaging?
1. What does experimenting mean to the patient?
2. Can the patient imagine doing this experiment?
3. Is there any part of this that the patient may need to practice with the clinician before the end of the visit?
4. What might get in the way of the patient *doing* the experiment?
5. Is the patient confident about *doing* the experiment? 1 is not at all confident and 10 is very confident
If not a 7 or higher in confidence ask, "How shall we change this to bring up your confidence?"
B. Is the experiment SMART?
☐ Specific
☐ Measurable
☐ Attainable
☐ Relevant to patient's values
☐ Timely

[a]SMART inspired by YourCoach, BVBA; https://www.yourcoach.be/en/coaching-tools/smart-goal-

Table D.5.4 Bull's-eye plan worksheet

1. Begin the conversation by asking what value seems most important as a guide for working with the problem. Ask the patient to talk more about that value, identifying a time in their life when that value inspired them. When they talk about the memory, slow the pace of the interview and encourage them to attend to thoughts and feelings that show up. Ask for more details. Often, patients will experience emotion and, if so, encourage them to allow it and use it to fuel actions they may want to take at this point in life.
2. Reflect on what you hear and then write a statement on the Bull's-Eye plan using words and images the patient used when talking about the value.
3. Explain that the bull's-eye on the target represents the strongest connection possible between a behavior representing a value and the experience of the value. Explain that the purpose of the bull's-eye is to direct our attention or focus. Most people do not hit the target. However, having a target helps us make daily choices with more awareness and attention.
4. Ask the patient to choose a number to represent how close to the bull's-eye value statement their behavior has come, on average, over the past 2 weeks (1 is outer circle and 7 is bull's-eye).
5. Ask the patient to plan a specific behavioral experiment to do in the next 2 weeks; one that they believe would tell that them they are on target and perhaps have moved closer to the bull's-eye than their average for the past 2 weeks.
6. If time allows, ask the patient to anticipate possible barrier(s) to their implementing the plan and teach a skill to help the patient work with an anticipated barrier. Barriers are often related to skill deficits in one or more of the pillars.
7. At follow-up, ask the patient to make a mark on the target to indicate consistency between behaviors and the targeted value. Discuss their experience with the plan. Identify barrier(s) to implementing the plan and teach skills that address the barrier(s). Then, plan another behavioral experiment to help the patient flourish.

Table D.5.5   Life path plan worksheet

1. How long have you had the problem that brings you here?
With this question, the clinician is inviting the patient to look at the problem from a different perspective, a view that encourages them to step back and look at their life over a longer period of time. The clinician might use the metaphor of an "eagles eye view versus a mouse view".
2. What have you tried? Helpful results? Less helpful results?
The clinician is attempting to identify the patient's efforts to solve the problem and how these efforts have impacted the problem and the patient's ability to flourish. Many times, patients have found ways to control or diminish difficult thoughts and feelings on a short-term basis. These strategies may have costs or unanticipated negative consequences. If so, what?
3. What do you want from life?
Here, the clinician is attempting to engage the patient in a conversation about the values that are most important at this moment in their life.
4. What are the barriers to doing what you want in life?
The clinician is attempting to help the patient identify reasons, rules and stories that play a role in maintaining the status quo. Patients may be able to hear themselves in a new way, as they recount reasons they've never questioned or tell stories that they may be able to experience now as old and automatic. The clinician might suggest that barriers may include things the patient is doing to avoid or control difficult feelings and thoughts.
5. What do you do when the barriers show up?
What most patients do when barriers show up is to control them (e.g., "try not to think about it" or "do something to distract myself").
6. Are you at war with the barriers? What are the consequences of being "at war" with the barriers?
When a patient is at war, they are probably using most of their resources for control and avoidance. They may be unable to connect with their values and see the possibility of more approach-oriented behavior. If this is the case, the clinician will try to help the patient find a way to "turn-around", even a little, so that a connection with values is possible, and to let the barriers come with them as they turn. The clinician will help the client have the barriers in a way that requires less effort and less struggle. The patient can learn to notice and name barriers rather than fight them, freeing energy for pursuing what matters.

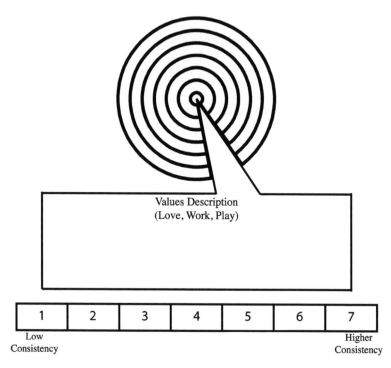

Fig. D.5.1   Bull's-eye plan

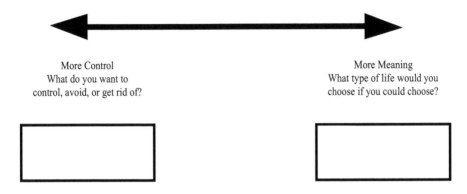

More Control
What do you want to
control, avoid, or get rid of?

More Meaning
What type of life would you
choose if you could choose?

1. Where are you on your life path? Mark an X. Which direction are you moving toward?

2. What, if any, are the costs and benefits of moving towards control?

3. Why would you want to move toward your values now? What values?

4. What behaviors would tell you that you're moving toward more meaning in life?

5. How would you turn in the direction of a more meaningful life?

6. When you turn toward control, how will you know to turn toward meaning?

7. Who or what helps you move in the direction of more meaning?

Fig. D.5.3 Life path plan. (Adapted from Strosahl, Robinson & Gustavsson, 2012 (Choosing: My Life Path and Turn-Around))

References

Agency for Healthcare Research and Quality. (2014). Defining the PCMH. http://www.pcmh.ahrq. gov. Accessed 14 June 2014. 30.

Altschuler, J., Margollus, D., Bodenheimer, T., & Grumbach, K. (2012). Estimating a reasonable patient panel size for primary care physicians with team-based task delegation. *Annals of Family Medicine, 10*(5), 396–400. https://doi.org/10.1370/afm.1400

American Association of Naturopathic Physicians. (2014). Accessed at http://www.naturopathic. org. Accessed 20 Aug 2014.

American Psychiatric Association. (2016). Diagnostic and statistical manual of mental disorders, (5thed.). (DSM-5), Washington, DC: American Psychological Association.

American Psychological Association Practice Association. (2009). Health care reform: Congress should ensure that psychologists' services are key in primary care initiatives. www.apapractice. org. Accessed 10 July 2013.

Auerbach, D. I., Chen, P. G., Friedberg, G. W., Reid, R. O., Lau, C., et al. (2013). Nurse-managed health centers and patient-centered medical homes could mitigate expected primary care physician shortage. *Health Affairs, 32*(11), 1933–1941.

Berwick, D. M., Nolan, T. W., & Whittington, J. (2008). The triple aim: Care, health and cost. *Health Affairs, 27*(3), 759–769.

Bodenheimer, T., & Sinsky, C. (2014). From triple to quadruple aim: Care of the patients requires care of the provider. *Annals of Family Medicine, 12*(6), 573–576. https://doi.org/10.1370/afm.1713

Bohlmeijer, E. T., Lamers, S. M. A., & Fledderus, M. (2015). Flourishing in people with depressive symptomatology increases with Acceptance and Commitment Therapy. Post-hoc analyses of a randomized controlled trial. *Behaviour Research and Therapy, 65*, 101–106. https://doi. org/10.1016/j.brat.2014.12.014

Bond, F. W., Hayes, S. C., Baer, R. A., Carpenter, K. M., Guenole, N., Orcutt, H. K., … Zettle, R. D. (2011). Preliminary psychometric properties of the Acceptance and Action Questionnaire – II: A revised measure of psychological inflexibility and experiential avoidance. *Behavior Therapy, 42*(4), 676–688. https://doi.org/10.1016/j.beth.2011.03.007

Cesene, D. F. (2016). Understanding the moderators of adverse childhood experiences on mature adult satisfaction and adjustment. Doctoral dissertation. Youngstown State University. OhioLINK ETD Center and the Maag Library Circulation Desk. Accessed 20 June 2019.

Ciarrochi, J., Hayes, l., & Bailey, A. (2012). *Get out of your mind and into your life or teens: A guide to living an extraordinary life.* Oakland, CA: New Harbinger.

© The Author(s), under exclusive license to Springer Nature
Switzerland AG Pte Ltd 2019
P. J. Robinson, *Basics of Behavior Change in Primary Care*, SpringerBriefs
in Psychology, https://doi.org/10.1007/978-3-030-32050-8

Cigrang, J. A., Rauch, S. A., Avila, L. L., Bryan, C. J., Goodie, J. L., Hryshko-Mullen, A., ... STRONG STAR Consortium. (2011). Treatment of active-duty military with PTSD in primary care: Early findings. *Psychological Services, 8*(2), 104–113.

Clark, D., Layard, R., Smithies, R., Richards, D., Suckling, R., & Wright, B. (2009). Improving access to psychological therapy: Initial evaluation of two UK demonstration sites. *Behaviour Research and Therapy, 47*, 910–920. https://doi.org/10.1371/journal.pone.0062873

Cooper, R. A. (2007). New directions for nurse practitioners and physician assistants in an era of physician shortages. *Academic Medicine, 82*(9), 827–828.

Coplan, B., Cawley, J., & Stoehr, J. (2013). Physician assistants in primary care: Trends and characteristics. *Annals of Family Medicine, 11*(1), 75–79.

Dindo, L. (2015). One-day Acceptance and Commitment training workshops in medical populations. *Current Opinions in Psychology, 2*, 38–42. https://doi.org/10.1016/jcopsye.2015.018.

Dobmeyer, A. E. (2018). *Psychological treatments of medical patients in integrated primary care* (Clinical Health Psychology Series). Washington, DC: American Psychological Association.

Dobson, K., Pusch, D, & Klassen, C. (2017). Workshop 2 – developing a Trauma-informed treatment in primary care: The embrace model for patients with adverse childhood experiences. Association for Behavioral and Cognitive Therapies, 2018.

Duke Family Medicine and Community Health Department. Duke health profile (DUKE), Duke health profile-8 (Duke-8) and the Duke population health profile (Duke-PH, for details see https://fmch.duke.edu/research/duke-health-measures.

Felitti, V. J., Anda, R. F., Nordenberg, D., Williamson, D. F., Spitz, A. M., Edwards, V., ... Marks, J. S. (1998). Relationship of childhood abuse and household dysfunction to many of the leading causes of death in adults. The Adverse Childhood Experiences (ACE) study. *American Journal of Preventive Medicine, 14*(4), 245–258.

Flaxman, P. E. & Bond, F. W. (2006). Acceptance and commitment therapy in the workplace. In Mindfulness-Based Treatment Approaches: https://doi.org/10.1016/B978-012088519-0/50018-6.

Flaxman, P. E., Bond, F. W., & Livheim, F. (2013). *The mindful and effective employee: An Acceptance and Commitment Therapy training manual for improving well-being and performance*. Oakland, CA: New Harbinger.

Fledderus, M., Bohlmeijer, E. T., Smit, F., & Westerhof, G. J. (2010). Mental health promotion as a new goal in public mental healthcare: A randomized controlled trial of an intervention enhancing psychological flexibility. *American Journal of Public Health, 100*, 2372–2378. https://doi.org/10.2105/AJPH.2010.196196

Frances, A. (2012) Two fallacies invalidate the DSM-5 field trials. *Psychiatric Times*, January 10, 2012. https://www.psychiatrictimes.com/dsm-5/two-fallacies-invalidate-dsm-5-field-trials. Accessed 20 June 2019.

Freeman, D. (2011). Blending behaviorists into the patient centered health care home. In N. A. Cummings & W. T. O'Donohue (Eds.), *Understanding the behavioral health care crisis: The promise of integrated care and diagnostic reform*. New York, NY: Routledge.

Gallimore, C., Corso, K. A., Robinson, P. J., & Runyan, C. N. (2018). Pharmacists in primary care: Lessons learned from integrated behavioral health. *Medical Practice Management*, 321–325.

Glover, N. G., Sylvers, P. D., Shearer, E. M., Kane, M.-C., Clasen, P. C., Epler, A. J., ... Bonow, J. T. (2016). The efficacy of focused acceptance and commitment therapy in VA primary care. *Psychological Services, 13*(2), 156–161.

Goodie, J., Isler, W., Hunter, C., & Peterson, A. (2009). Using behavioral health consultants to treat insomnia in primary care: A clinical case series. *Journal of Clinical Psychology, 65*, 294–304.

Hayes, S. C. ACT and the core design principles. https://www.prosocial.world/post/act-and-the-core-design-principles. Accessed 6 Dec 2019.

Hayes, S. C., Luoma, J. B., Bond, F. W., Masuda, A., & Lillis, J. (2006). Acceptance and commitment therapy: Model, processes and outcomes. *Behavior Research and Therapy, 44*(1), 1–25.

Hayes, S. C., & Smith, S. (2005). *Get out of your mind and into your life: The new acceptance and commitment therapy*. Oakland, CA: New Harbinger.

Hayes, S. C., Strosahl, K. D., & Wilson, K. G. (2012). Acceptance and commitment therapy. In *The process and practice of mindful change* (2nd ed.). New York, NY: Guilford.

Herrman, H. S, Saxena, S., Moodie, R. (Eds.) (2005). Promoting mental health: Concepts, emerging evidence, practice. A WHO report in collaboration with the Victorian Health Promotion Foundation and the University of Melbourne. Geneva: World Health Organization. Available at: http://www.who.int/mental_health/evi-dence/MH_Promotion_Book.pdf. Accessed 22 Jan 2010.

Hoff, T., Weller, W., & DePuccio, M. (2012). The patient-centered medical home: A review of recent research. *Medical Care Research and Review, 69*(6), 619–644.

Hunter, C. L., Funderburk, J. S., Polaha, J., Bauman, D., Goodie, J. L., & Hunter, C. M. (2017a). Primary Care Behavioral Health (PCBH) model research: Current state of the science and a call to action. *Journal of Clinical Psychology in Medical Settings*. https://doi.org/10.1007/s10880-017-9512-0

Hunter, C. L., Goodie, J. L., Oordt, M. S., & Dobmeyer, A. C. (2017b). *Integrated behavioral health in primary care: Step-by-step guidance for assessment and intervention* (2nd ed.). Washington, DC: American Psychological Association.

Huppert, F. A., & So, T. T. C. (2009). What percentage of people in Europe are flourishing and what characterizes them? Prepared for the OECD/ISQOLS meeting "Measuring subjective well-being: An opportunity for NSOs?", Florence, July 23–24, 2009. http://citeseerx.ist.psu.edu/viewdoc/download? Accessed 21 June 2019. 10.1.1.550.8290&rep=rep1&type=pdf.

Institute of Medicine of the National Academies. (1996, January 01). Primary Care: America's Health in a New Era. Washington, DC: Institute of Medicine. http://www.iom.edu/CMS/3809/27706.aspx. Accessed 23 June 2005.

John, J. R., Ghassempour, S., Girosi, F., & Atlantis, E. (2018). The effectiveness of patient—centered medical home model versus standard primary care in chronic disease management: protocol for a systematize review and meta-analysis of randomized and non—randomized controlled trials. *BioMed Central Systematic Reviews, 7*, 215. https://doi.org/10.1186/s13643-018-0887-2

Kashdan, T., & Rottenberg, J. (2010). Psychological flexibility as a fundamental aspect of health. *Clinical Psychology Review, 30*(7), 865–878. https://doi.org/10.1016/j.cpr.2010.03.001

Katon, W., Robinson, P., Von Korff, M., Lin, E., Bush, T., et al. (1996). A multifaceted intervention to improve treatment of depression in primary care. *Archives of General Psychiatry, 53*, 924–932.

Keyes, C. L. (2009). The black-white paradox in health: Flourishing in the face of social inequality and discrimination. *Journal of Personality, 77*(6), 1677–1706. https://doi.org/10.1111/j.1467-6494.2009.00597.x

Keyes, C. L. M., & Haidt, J. (2013). *Flourishing: Positive psychology and the life well lived*. Washington, DC: American Psychological Association.

Maryland Department of Housing and Community Development. 2016. EmPOWER maryland low income energy efficiency program. Accessed 2016 June 14.

Maslach, C., Schaufell, W. B., & Leiter, M. P. (2001). Job burnout. *Annual Review of Psychology, 52*, 397–422. https://doi.org/10.1146/annurev.psych.52.1.397

Maslach, C., & Jackson, S. (2018). The Maslach Burnout Inventory – Human Services Survey for Medical Personnel (MBI-HSS (MP). Available on line: https://www.mindgarden.com/mbi-human-services-survey-medical-personnel/698-mbihssmp-individual-report.html.

Minnesota Housing Finance Agency. (2016). Rehabilitation loan/emergency and accessibility loan program. Accessed 14 June 2016.

Olfson, M., Mojitabai, R., Sampson, N., Hwang, I., & Kessler, R. (2009). Dropout from outpatient mental healthcare in the United States. *Psychiatric Services, 60*, 898–907. https://doi.org/10.1176/ps.2009.60.7.898

Peikes, D., Zutshi, A., Genevro, J. L., Parchman, M. L., & Meyers, D. S. (2012). Early evaluations of the medical home: Building on a promising start. *American Journal of Managed Care, 18*(2), 105–116.

Poole, J. C., Dobson, K. S., & Pusch, D. (2017). Childhood adversity and adult depression: The protective role of psychological resilience. *Child Abuse & Neglect, 64*, 89–100. https://doi.org/10.1016/j.chiabu.2016.12

Radkrahishnan, R., Hammond, G., Jones, P., Watson, A., McMillan-Shields, F., & LaFortune, S. (2013). Costs of the Improving Access to Psychological Therapies (IAPT) programme: An analysis of cost of session, treatment and recovery in selected primary care trusts in the East of England. *Behaviour Research and Therapy, 51*, 37–45. https://doi.org/10.1016/j.brat.2012.10.001

Reid, R. J., Coleman, K., Johnson, E. A., Fishman, P. A., Hsu, C., et al. (2010, May). The group health medical home at year two: Cost savings, higher patient satisfaction, and less burnout for providers. *Health Affairs, 29*(5), 835–843. https://doi.org/10.1377/hlthaff.2010.0158.

Reiter, J. T., Dobmeyer, A. C., & Hunter, C. L. (2017). The primary care behavioral health (PCBH) model: An overview and operational definition. *Journal of Clinical Psychology in Medical Settings, 24*(4). National Committee for Quality Assurance 2011.

Robinson, P., Bush, T., Von Korff, M., Katon, W., Lin, E., et al. (1995). Primary care physician use of cognitive behavioral techniques with depressed patients. *Journal of Family Practice, 40*(4), 352–357.

Robinson, P. J., & Reiter, J. D. (2007). *Behavioral consultation and primary care: A guide to integrating services.* New York, NY: Springer.

Robinson, P. J., & Reiter, J. D. (2015). *Behavioral consultation and primary care: A guide to integrating services* (2nd ed.). New York, NY: Springer.

Robinson, P. J., Gould, D., & Strosahl, K. D. (2010). *Real behavior change in primary care. Strategies and tools for improving outcomes and increasing job satisfaction.* Oakland, CA: New Harbinger.

Robinson, P. J., Oyemaja, J., Beachy, B., Goodie, J., Bell, J., Sprague, L., … Ward, C. (2018). Creating a primary care workforce: Strategies for leaders, clinicians, and nurses. *Journal of Clinical Psychology in Medical Settings, 20*(3). https://doi.org/10.1007/s10880-017-9530-y

Robinson, P. Von Korff, M., Bush, T., Lin, E. H. B., & Ludman, E. J. (submitted). The impact of primary care behavioral health services on patient behaviors: A randomized controlled trial.

Rosenthal, T. C. (2008). The medical home: Growing evidence to support a new approach to primary care. *Journal of the American Board of Family Medicine, 21*(5), 427–440.

Schotanus-Dijkstra, M., ten Have, M., Lamers, S. M. A., de Graaf, R., & Bohlmeijer, E. T. (2017). The longitudinal relationship between flourishing mental health and mood, anxiety and substance use disorders. *European Journal of Public Health, 27*(3), 563–568. https://doi.org/10.1093/eurpub/ckw202

Seligman, M. E. P. (2012). *Flourish: A visionary new understanding of happiness and well-being.* New York, NY: Simon & Schuster.

Siefel, M., & Nolan, K. (2012). A guide to measuring the triple aim: Population health, experience of care, and per capita cost. IHI Innovation Series white paper. Cambridge, MA: Institute for Healthcare Improvement; 2012. http://www.IHI.org. Accessed 6 June 2014. SMART https://www.yourcoach.be/en/coaching-tools/smart-goal-setting.php.

Soots, L. (2018). The positive psychology people. http://www.thepositivepsychologypeople.com/flourishing/. Accessed 18 June 2019.

Starfield, B. (2008). Refocusing the system. *New England Journal of Medicine, 359*, 2087–2091.

Starfield, B., Shi, L., & Macinko. (2005). Contribution of primary care to health systems and health. *The Millbank Quarterly: A Multidisplinary Journal of Population Health and Health Policy, 83*(3), 457–502.

Stoddard, J. A., & Afari, N. (2014). *The big book of metaphors: A practitioner's guide to experiential exercises and metaphors in acceptance and commitment therapy.* Oakland, CA: New Harbinger.

Strosahl, K. D., Robinson, P. J., & Gustavsson, T. (2012). *Brief interventions for radical change: Principles and practice of focused acceptance and commitment therapy.* Oakland, CA: New Harbinger.

Strosahl, K. D., & Robinson, P. J. (2018). Adapting empirically supported treatments in the Era of integrated care: A roadmap for success. *Clinical Psychology: Science and Practice*. https://doi.org/10.1111/cpsp.12246

Swift, J., & Greenberg, R. (2012). Pre-mature discontinuation in adult psychotherapy: A meta-analysis. *Journal of Consulting and Clinical Psychology, 80*, 547–559. https://doi.org/10.1037/a0028226

U.S. Department of Agriculture. Rural development. Single family housing repair loans & grants 2016. Available from: Single Family Housing Repair Loans & Grants. Accessed 14 June 2016.

United States Department of Health. Office of disease prevention and health promotion. Healthy People 2020. https://www.healthypeople.gov Accessed 20 June 2019.

Van derWeele, T. J. (2017). On the promotion of human flourishing. *Proceedings of the National Academy of Sciences USA, 31*, 8148–8156.

Index

© The Author(s), under exclusive license to Springer Nature
Switzerland AG Pte Ltd 2019
P. J. Robinson, *Basics of Behavior Change in Primary Care*, SpringerBriefs
in Psychology, https://doi.org/10.1007/978-3-030-32050-8